SIMPLY NUTRITIOUS!

Recipes and Recommendations to Reduce Your Risk of Cancer

Sabine M. Artaud-Wild, R.D.
Editor

American Cancer Society
Oregon Division, Inc.
Portland, Oregon

Recipes in this book have been collected from various sources and tested by volunteers for the American Cancer Society, Oregon Division, Inc. We believe that following instructions found in this book will produce successful results. Ingredients and cooking procedures, however, vary greatly, so cooks should not hesitate to question or test before preparation. Neither the American Cancer Society, Oregon Division, Inc., nor any contributor is responsible for cooking results that may not prove satisfactory.

This book is published to enhance the health of its readers and persons for whom they buy and cook food. Any portion of it may be reproduced for non-commercial use without permission from the publisher. When making such reproductions, please cite this book as the source.

Reproduction in any form of any portion of this book for commercial purposes requires prior written permission from the publisher.

Published and copyright 1986 by
American Cancer Society
Oregon Division, Inc.
0330 SW Curry Street
Portland OR 97201

Printed and bound in the USA

Library of Congress Cataloging in Publication Data
Artaud-Wild, Sabine M., ed., date
Simply Nutritious!
Rev. ed. of: Simply nutritious / Sabine Artaud-Wild, 1985.
Bibliography: p.
Includes index.
1. Cancer—Diet therapy—Recipes. 2. Cancer—Diet therapy.
3. Cancer—Prevention. I. Artaud-Wild, Sabine M. II. Artaud-Wild, Sabine
M. Simply Nutritious. III. American Cancer Society. Oregon Division.
[DNLM: 1. Diet—popular works. 2. Neoplasms—prevention &
control—popular works. QZ 201 S612]
RC271.D52S56   1986   616.99'405   86-71576
ISBN 0-9617128-1-3 (kitchen binding)
ISBN 0-9617128-0-5 (library binding)

FOREWORD

There is no diet known that will cure cancer; nor is there yet proof that cancer can be prevented by changing our diet. So why is the American Cancer Society producing this recipe book? This book is being written now because convincing evidence is accumulating that some of the most common cancers in the United States may be related to the diet we consume; and that changing the food we eat and share with our families may reduce the risk of getting one of those cancers in the future. The changes recommended are simple, not expensive, and can be fun.

The people of the United States—and other industrialized nations —consume a diet high in fat from all sources, including cream, butter, margarine, meat, cheese, and eggs. Grains and carbohydrates are often refined by removing fiber-containing husks (bran), reducing the beneficial complex carbohydrates to refined ones with less nutritional value. In addition, many of our prepared foods, such as pastries, luncheon meats, hotdogs, granola bars, and potato chips, contain large amounts of hidden fat. In other areas of the world, people consume a diet high in fish, whole grains, legumes, and vegetables, resulting in lower fat and higher roughage (fiber) intakes.

Whereas cancer of the breast, uterus, prostate and colon are leading causes of cancer death here, they are much less common in those areas. Japan is a country with a fat intake only half that of the United States. Japan has an incidence of breast cancer that is half that of the United States and until after World War II had almost no cancer of the prostate. When a Japanese family moved to the United States and adopted our type of diet, their descendants developed these cancers as frequently as other native born Americans. Extra fat in the diet increases the risk of getting heart disease, but serves as a nucleus for the synthesis of certain hormones that can stimulate the growth of cancer of the breast, prostate, and uterus.

Colon cancer begins in the lining of the large intestine. It may be started by cancer-causing chemicals (carcinogens) that have prolonged contact with the lining. One potent carcinogen, fecopentaene, is produced by certain bacteria in the intestine. The quantity produced is much less when fiber is added to the diet. In addition, fiber stimulates the intestines to move the contents more rapidly and thus to reduce the time of exposure. Other carcinogens in food may evolve from nitrites that are used as additives, and nitrosamines produced by smoking and charring of food.

Increased alcohol consumption is associated with cancer of the liver, and in smokers, is associated with increased cancers of the mouth, throat, pharynx and esophagus.

As a medical oncologist, I am often asked what diet I would recommend for healthy people. A good diet now would reduce the total amount of fats from the current 40% of total calories eaten to under 30%. It would restore much of the natural fiber in our foods by replacing white flour with whole grains and increasing the total fiber intake to one to two ounces daily. High fat desserts and prepared foods would become occasional treats. Smoked and nitrite-cured foods would be avoided when possible. Alcohol consumption would be restricted. The diet changes included in this book are not only sensible for reducing the risk of cancer, but fit the recommended guidelines for preventing that other big killer in America, coronary heart disease.

William P. Galen, M.D.
Oregon Medical Delegate to American Cancer Society
Past President, Oregon Division, American Cancer Society

PREFACE

In 1984 the American Cancer Society issued a series of dietary guidelines to help reduce the risk of developing cancer. Although no concrete dietary advice can guarantee the prevention of cancer, there is enough scientific evidence to recommend some prudent food choices to the American public.

Twenty years ago, an association of smoking and lung cancer was reported by scientists, but the link could not be established with complete certainty. A warning was given in cautious wording out of scientific probity. Today the link is clearly established and the recommendation to stop smoking to avoid lung cancer is unequivocal. We now know that many deaths could have been prevented if Americans could have been persuaded to stop smoking. We are now in a similar interim phase with dietary warnings. It may be too soon to make firm recommendations, but interim guidelines make sense.

In response to the American Cancer Society's dietary guidelines, the Oregon Division of the Society published a cookbook explaining the role of diet in cancer prevention and providing recipes based on the Society's recommendations. We received such a favorable response to that first book that we decided to produce this revised edition. We have updated and clarified dietary information, revised the original recipes where needed, and added new recipes. We hope that this new book will promote healthful eating habits while raising the dollars necessary to support the American Cancer Society programs of research, education, and service.

The interest and hard work of many people made the idea for this project become a reality and have made possible this revised edition. Numerous volunteers and organizations contributed recipes. A list of these contributors appears after the recipes. Dietitians Deanna Voytilla, R.D., and Charles Slaughter, R.D., helped with the recipe testing. We also want to thank the dedicated members of our committee, who divided the recipes among themselves to test and taste them. We would like to specially thank Sabine Artaud-Wild, R.D., for her time and effort in creating the text of this book. Our appreciation also goes to Portland, Oregon, artist Sally Haley for the use of her painting on the cover.

We hope that readers find *Simply Nutritious!* a useful source of nutritional guidance and creative recipes for an eating style to reduce the risk of cancer and maintain overall health.

Susan Schnitzer
Chair

CONTENTS

TABLES

INTRODUCTION

Simply Nutritious! is a cookbook—and more. From appetizers to desserts, you will find recipes to attract the eye and tempt the palate. You will also find the reasons for the American Cancer Society dietary guidelines these recipes follow. And you will learn about ways to adopt a cancer prevention diet not only at home but at work, when eating out, or while traveling.

Simply Nutritious! tells about research into the role of diet in cancer prevention and explains the American Cancer Society's interim dietary guidelines. You will also find descriptions of the food groups basic to good health and information about how a cancer prevention diet balances these food groups.

To help with the adoption of such an eating style, we give pointers on how to select, buy, and prepare food. Tables and charts show the amount of fat in various foods, which ones to select, which to use less often, and how to use them. Information is given about various cooking methods. Tips are included for snacking and for eating out.

Following the list of recipe contributors are further notes on cancer prevention and a list of other publications you may find useful.

As you read this book you will see that a cancer prevention style of eating is not a diet in the usual sense, but part of a way of living to lessen the risk of cancer and maintain good health. When this style of eating is a habit, you can afford your favorite high fat, high calorie entrée or dessert on occasion. The old rule—everything in moderation—still holds. It is a fitting motto for a cancer prevention style of eating.

We are proud of *Simply Nutritious!* We think you will find the information and recipes a great help in developing and following a healthful diet that will help reduce the risk of cancer.

RESEARCH ON CANCER PREVENTION

There is reason for hope and optimism in cancer prevention. Hope comes from the massive effort made by scientists to determine the factors responsible for the development of cancer and to find ways to prevent it. Optimism comes from research on the influence of environmental factors such as life style, workplace hazards, and diet on the development of cancer.

The results of this research have led many scientists to believe that environmental factors are as influential as heredity in cancer formation. These findings suggest that a great number of cancers could be prevented, and so the optimism: while ancestry cannot be changed, a lot can be done to alter environment.

ROLE OF DIET

Poor diet is thought to be one of the most important environmental risk factors in the development of human cancer. While many of us think of poor diet as obtaining too little of the nutrients essential to good health, overconsumption can also be a factor. Ironically, malnutrition can be a penalty of abundance.

Much of what has been learned about the role of diet in the formation of cancers has come from the studies of populations (epidemiology). These studies show that the incidence of cancers differs greatly among countries and among groups within countries. In the United States, cancers of the breast, uterus, prostate, and colon are the leading causes of cancer death. These cancers are much less common in some other coun-

3

tries. While the specific cause and effect relationships remain uncertain, there is evidence that some of these cancers may be related to our diet.

One study of populations compared diet and incidence of cancers in Japan and the United States. Japanese consume only about half as much fat as do people in the United States. The study showed that the incidence of breast cancer in Japan is half that of the United States. The research also showed that Japanese who emigrated to Hawaii, the United States, or Canada and adopted a diet similar to that of the host countries developed cancer patterns closer to people born in the host countries than to Japanese who remained in their home country.

Evidence of a link between diet and cancer also comes from laboratory experiments on rats or mice and on cells. These experiments confirm the association of certain eating habits with the development of various cancers, mostly those of the gastrointestinal tract and of the breast, uterus, and prostate.

Cause and effect relationships between diet and cancer are difficult to pinpoint. The reasons are many. For example, some foods contain substances which can cause tumors, while other foods contain some natural inhibitors of the process which leads to the full development of cancerous tumors.

More research on the development of cancer in the body must be done before scientists can say that a particular substance causes or promotes a specific cancer. We do know, however, that cancer develops in two main steps. A change in normal cells is caused by an initiator. The transformed cell is susceptible to environmental influences, or promoters of cancer. Diet is considered a possible promoter of cancer rather than an initiator. Ongoing research will help elucidate this role.

DIETARY GUIDELINES

Although at present there is no diet that can be said to guarantee the prevention of any specific human cancer, the American Cancer Society believes there is sufficient information to warrant recommendations about nutrition. These guidelines are similar to statements previously issued by the Society, the National Research Council of the National

Academy of Sciences, and the National Cancer Institute. Because the recommendations will be updated as research continues, they are referred to as "interim" guidelines.

The Society's dietary guidelines have been developed not only with cancer prevention in mind, but in the interests of the maintenance of good health. These recommendations generally conform with the U.S. Dietary Guidelines for Americans issued in 1980 by the U.S. Department of Agriculture and the then U.S. Department of Health, Education and Welfare, and the guidelines of the American Heart Association and the American Diabetes Association.

The American Cancer Society is currently conducting a six-year project—the Cancer Prevention Study II—to examine the lives, eating habits, work, and environmental exposures of 1.2 million Americans. It is hoped that this study will establish new positive and negative links between diet, nutrition, and cancer.

In addition, the American Cancer Society is supporting numerous grants in nutrition research. These and other investigations in this country and abroad should provide more definite answers to the questions: What causes cancer? What is the exact role of diet in cancer? What is the best way to prevent cancer? In the meantime, the American Cancer Society offers interim dietary guidelines to help you and your family follow a diet consistent with current knowledge on the dietary prevention of cancer.

AMERICAN CANCER SOCIETY
INTERIM DIETARY GUIDELINES

Simply stated, the American Cancer Society Interim Dietary Guidelines mean an eating style low in fat, high in fiber, rich in foods from plant sources, and with small amounts of foods from low fat animal sources (dairy products, meats, and fats). In considering such an eating style, it is important to know the what and why of the recommendations. Here are the Interim Dietary Guidelines and their bases.

1. AVOID OBESITY

The American Cancer Society's massive study of almost a million people, Cancer Prevention Study I, conducted from 1960 to 1972, found an increased incidence of cancer of the gallbladder, kidney, stomach, colon, breast, and lining of the uterus in obese people. In that study men and women 40% overweight had a greater risk of cancer than those with normal weight. Studies in animals show that their risk of cancer is reduced and their life span increased when they are fed a diet which maintains an ideal weight.

Obesity is associated with changes in the metabolism of hormones. There may be a link between body weight, hormone levels, and risk of cancer. Thus the American Cancer Society recommends that everyone reach and maintain an ideal weight through appropriate eating and increased exercise.

2. CUT DOWN ON TOTAL FAT INTAKE

Fat is the substance for which there is the strongest evidence of a link between diet and cancer. Studies of human populations suggest that a high intake of fat increases the risk of colon, breast, and prostate cancers. Experimental studies in rats also have shown that high fat diets increase the incidence of cancers of the breast and colon in those animals exposed to carcinogens (cancer producing substances).

Animal research indicates a distinction between the effects of polyunsaturated and saturated fats on tumor production when total fat intake is low, polyunsaturates being the more cancer producing, but not when total fat intake is high. Information from human cancer studies does not allow such a clear distinction to be made. Excessive intake of all fats, both saturated and unsaturated, whether from plant or animal sources, increases the development of breast, colon, and prostate cancers. Besides, diets high in fat are also high in calories. Cutting down on fat will help in preventing obesity.

Americans consume about 40% of their calories as fat. The American Cancer Society recommends that fat consumption be reduced to no more than 30% of total calories.

3. EAT MORE HIGH FIBER FOODS

A high fiber diet may protect against colon cancer. Fiber, also known as roughage, refers to a number of substances not readily digested in the intestines. It is a complex mixture of components such as cellulose, lignin, gums, pectins, and mucilages. These are found in unrefined grains, bran, legumes, fruits, and vegetables. It is not known which substance is most helpful in reducing the risk of cancer.

The exact role of fiber in cancer prevention has not yet been established nor is agreement about this role universally recognized. Early populations studies showed that colorectal cancer is low in populations who live on a diet of largely unrefined food which is high in fiber. One animal study reported no association between high total fiber intake and a lower risk of colon cancer but a protective effect of one of the fiber components. This component is found mostly in whole wheat products and bran. Other studies have indicated that the consumption of cellulose and bran prevents the development of colon cancer induced by chemical carcinogens.

In any case, a refined diet low in fiber is likely to be a high fat one. Even if fiber by itself does not protect against cancer, high fiber containing cereals, legumes, fruits, and vegetables are excellent choices to replace fatty foods. The American Cancer Society recommends a liberal intake of these fiber-containing foods.

4. INCLUDE FOODS RICH IN VITAMIN A AND C

Deep yellow and dark green vegetables as well as yellow orange fruits are rich in beta carotene. Beta carotene is a form, or precursor, of vitamin A; it is converted into vitamin A by the body. Studies indicate that food rich in vitamin A and beta carotene may lower the risk of cancer of the larynx, esophagus, and lung.

However, because vitamin A is fat soluble and is stored in the liver, it is toxic in large quantities. The American Cancer Society recommends that vitamin A come from natural sources rather than from vitamin pills.

Although there is still a great deal of controversy about it, some studies have shown that consumption of foods high in vitamin C, or ascorbic acid, is associated with a lower risk of developing cancer of the esophagus and stomach. Vitamin C can inhibit the formation in the stomach of cancer-producing nitrosamines and also help maintain the strength of the immune system of the body.

The American Cancer Society recommends eating fruits and vegetables rich in vitamins A and C liberally—at least five servings a day.

5. INCLUDE CRUCIFEROUS VEGETABLES

Broccoli, Brussels sprouts, cabbage, cauliflower, and kale belong to the mustard family and are members of a large group of vegetables called cruciferous. Cruciferous vegetables derive their name from the special pattern of their flowers whose four petals are in the shape of a cross—the Latin word is crux.

There are substances in these vegetables which appear to protect against cancer of the gastrointestinal and respiratory tracts. They inhibit the development of cancer in laboratory animals. It has not yet been determined which of these substances is protective.

The American Cancer Society recommends including broccoli, Brussels sprouts, cabbage, cauliflower, and kale in the daily diet. While not always among the favorite of Americans, these vegetables can be prepared in a number of interesting ways. In this recipe book we include a number of recipes using these cruciferous vegetables.

6. EAT MODERATELY OF SALT-CURED, SMOKED, AND NITRITE-CURED FOODS

Salt curing and smoking are methods used to preserve such foods as meats, fish, and sausages. Incomplete combustion in the smoking process results in tars, which are absorbed into the food. These tars contain carcinogens similar to tars in tobacco smoke. People in China, Japan, and Iceland who consume salt-cured, salt-pickled, or smoked food develop a great number of cancers of the stomach and the esophagus.

In addition, nitrites are commonly used to cure meats and fish to preserve their color and prevent botulism (food poisoning). In the body, nitrites can combine with protein to form nitrosamines. The U.S. Department of Agriculture and the meat industry have decreased the amount of nitrites added to cured meat. The food processing industry is now using a liquid smoke which is thought to be less hazardous.

The American Cancer Society recommends reducing or avoiding entirely the consumption of salt-cured, smoked, and nitrite-cured foods such as luncheon meats. Many of these foods are also high in fat.

7. KEEP ALCOHOL CONSUMPTION MODERATE, IF YOU DRINK

Excessive alcohol intake, especially when combined with cigarette smoking, increases the risk of cancer of the mouth, larynx, and esophagus. Population studies in Africa, China, and France show that the consumption of wine and other alcohols is linked with the development of cancers of the esophagus and liver.

While the American Cancer Society advises to reduce the consumption of alcohol, it does not prescribe any specific amount. Physicians and dietitians generally suggest that no more than two drinks be consumed per day. This advice is consistent with overall health protection.

Two drinks means two 12-ounce beers or two 4-ounce glasses of wine or two cocktails or any combination of two drinks. Physicians and dietitians do not recommend that two drinks be consumed every day, only that people who habitually drink limit their consumption to two drinks. The American Cancer Society recommends that if you drink, you do so in moderation.

OTHER NUTRITIONAL FACTORS

In a February 1984 report, *Nutrition and Cancer: Cause and Prevention*, the American Cancer Society made a number of additional comments about nutritional factors.

Food additives: Those additives which have been found to cause cancer already are banned. Some others may protect against the disease. A great deal of research is needed about the possible cancer risks or benefits of food additives before specific recommendations can be made.

Vitamin E: There is no evidence that vitamin E prevents cancer in humans, although antioxidants such as vitamin E have been shown to prevent some cancers in animal research.

Selenium: Evidence that selenium protects against some cancers is much too limited to justify recommendings its use. Because of the danger of selenium poisoning, the American Cancer Society warns against medically unsupervised use of selenium as a food supplement.

Artificial sweeteners: The long-term effects of new non-caloric sweeteners now entering the market have not yet been studied. Although high levels of saccharin have been shown to cause bladder cancer in rats, there is no clear evidence that its moderate use causes cancer in humans, except possibly in children and pregnant women.

Coffee: Although some epidemiologic studies implicate heavy coffee drinking in bladder and pancreas cancers, others have failed to do so. There is no indication at this time that caffeine, a component of both coffee and tea, is a risk factor in human cancer.

Meat and fish cooked at high temperatures, such as by frying or broiling: Some methods of smoking and cooking food at high temperatures, such as charcoal broiling, may result in mutagens forming and being deposited on the food. Mutagens are substances that cause changes in the genetic makeup of cells and are suspected to lead to cancer. The subject is being studied further.

Cholesterol: Evidence relating both high and low blood cholesterol levels to human cancer is inconclusive.

NOT A FAD DIET

The American Cancer Society entitles its Interim Dietary Guidelines brochure *Nutrition, Common Sense and Cancer.* As the title and the guidelines themselves indicate, the eating style recommended is not just another fad diet. The recommendations mean maintaining an appropriate weight while eating a well-balanced diet low in fat, high in fiber, with plenty of foods rich in vitamins A and C as well as some broccoli, Brussels sprouts, cauliflower, cabbage, or kale, and reducing salt-cured, smoked food and alcohol consumption. No quick-fix, no excess of one type of food, no total dietary exclusions, no unnecessary supplements.

HEALTHFUL EATING

You have decided to adopt a different life style. You want to follow a prudent way of eating, one which will lessen your chances of developing some forms of cancer and keep you in good health. At the same time, you do not want to be on a diet. Eating is one of life's greatest pleasures and you want to continue enjoying good food and flavorful dishes. Can you have both wishes? Yes. To help you get started—and continue—an eating style that features healthful, tasty food we present the following information. All the recipes are based on the principles discussed.

HOW MUCH OF WHAT?

A healthful eating style:

- Contains no more than 30% of calories from fats, as compared with the typical American diet containing more than 40%;

- Contains about 55% of calories from carbohydrates, as compared to 40-45% in a typical American diet;

- Stresses complex carbohydrates (starches and sugars occurring naturally, as in fruit);

- Contains at least 30 grams of dietary fiber per day as a result of an increased consumption of complex carbohydrates, as compared to an estimated 20 grams in the typical American diet;

- Contains a reasonable amount of protein, about 15% of calories, with an emphasis on vegetable proteins and low fat animal proteins;

- Provides the calories necessary to meet all the body's energy needs and maintain a desirable body weight but no more; and

- Includes foods rich in vitamins A and C.

BALANCING YOUR DIET

Foods are divided into groups according to the nutrients they contain. No single type of food can supply all the nutrients needed for a balanced diet. The more varied the food intake the better the chances of getting all the carbohydrates, proteins, fats, vitamins, and minerals needed to maintain good health.

Vegetables

Vegetables contain virtually no fat. They are also very low in calories, making them ideally suited for controlling weight. Vegetables are excellent sources of vitamins, particularly vitamins A and C, folacin, and vitamin B6, and contain a wealth of minerals. Dark green and deep yellow vegetables are especially rich in beta carotene—a building block for vitamin A, iron, calcium, magnesium, potassium, and zinc. As mentioned in the Interim Dietary Guidelines, some vegetables of the mustard family, such as broccoli, cauliflower, and cabbage, are thought to prevent some cancers. In addition, all vegetables contain complex carbohydrates and fiber. They should be eaten liberally—at least three servings a day, raw or cooked. If you cook them, remember that the shorter the cooking time, generally the more nutrients remain and the greater the color and taste.

Fruits

Like vegetables, most fruits contain no fat, provide fiber and carbohydrates, and are invaluable for their vitamin and mineral content. Many fruits contribute potassium to the diet, especially apricots, bananas, grapefruit, melons, grapes, and peaches. Fruit can satisfy a sweet tooth with very few calories and often has more nutrients than baked desserts. It is best to eat fruit raw and unpeeled, when possible, in order to consume all available fiber. Similarly, whole fruits are preferable to their juices: juices contain far less fiber and are higher in calories.

A word of caution: avocados and olives are higher in fat than most fruits. It is best to consume them in small quantities.

Grains

All cereals (including breakfast cereals), breads, rices, pastas, bulgur, semolina, couscous grain, kasha, flours, and bran products are grains. These are excellent sources of complex carbohydrates, iron, magnesium, zinc, calcium, protein, and thiamin and niacin. Whole grains and bran products have more fiber, folacin, and vitamin E than refined grains. They should be eaten liberally—at least six servings a day.

Contrary to a generally held belief, grains are not high in calories themselves and contain little fat. The fats, meats, or cheeses added to grain dishes are high in calories.

A word of caution: both commercially produced and homemade baked grain products such as crackers and cookies may contain a lot of fat. (See the table "Selecting Commercial Products.")

Legumes

This group includes all dried beans, lentils, dried peas, and tofu. Legumes are a good source of protein, yet contain no cholesterol and virtually no fat. They provide protein, fiber, complex carbohydrates, iron, magnesium, zinc, calcium, and many vitamins. A healthful eating style includes a variety of legumes weekly.

Nuts and Seeds

These foods are sources of protein, phosphorous, potassium, and some B vitamins. As members of the plant world, nuts and seeds contain no cholesterol. But they contain a lot of fat, and are very high in calories as a result. While they provide variety in texture to the diet, they properly belong to the fat group and should be used very sparingly. Especially high in fat are pecans and macadamia nuts. (See Nuts and Seeds in the table "Fat Content of Various Foods.")

Dairy Products

Dairy products include a variety of foods made from the milk of cows and goats. They are excellent sources of protein, calcium, phosphorous, magnesium, and vitamins A, D, folacin, riboflavin, and B12. However, whole milk (3.8-5% fat) and dairy products such as butter and cheese made from whole milk are high in fat and cholesterol. To get the nutritional benefits of these foods without the high fat and cholesterol, choose only low fat dairy products, including low fat cheeses. Cheeses as low as 1% or 2% fat are available. (See Milk Products and Cheeses in the table "Fat Content of Various Foods.")

Animal Protein Sources

All fish, shellfish, poultry, meats, eggs, organ meats, and dairy products are animal proteins. The non-dairy animal proteins provide substantial amounts of protein, iron, phosphorous, zinc, and B vitamins. Since many animal products are very high in fat and contain a lot of cholesterol, foods in this group have to be chosen judiciously. Happily, fish and shellfish are very low in fat. They are the animal protein food of choice. Poultry and rabbit come next. (See Fish, Shellfish, Poultry, Meats and also Luncheon Meats in the table "Fat Content of Various Foods.")

Decreasing animal protein in the diet should not be a matter of concern in terms of adequacy of protein intake. Foods besides meat, poultry, fish, and whole milk dairy products provide important amounts of protein. A diet that combines whole grains, legumes, fruits, and vegetables and reasonable amounts of low fat animal products can provide the daily intake of 45 grams of protein for women and 56 grams for men recommended by the Food and Nutrition Board of the National Academy of Sciences. The table "Protein" illustrates how easy it is to get more than the basic protein needs of the average adult.

Fats and Oils

Fats and oils may make food taste better. Butter and margarine are good sources of vitamins A and D. Vegetable oils provide vitamin E in good amounts. However, ounce for ounce, fats and oils provide over two times as many calories as proteins and carboydrates do: 9 calories per

---

PROTEIN

SOURCE	SERVINGS	GRAMS
Poultry, fish, lean meat	1 (4 oz., cooked)	28
Low fat dairy products	2	16
	Examples of 1 serving:	
	1 cup low fat milk	
	8 oz. low fat yogurt	
	¼ cup low fat cottage cheese	
	1 oz. part skim mozzarella	
Cereals, legumes, bread, starchy foods	5	15
	Examples of 1 serving:	
	1½ slices whole wheat bread	
	¾ cup bran	
	¾ cup cooked beans	
	1 large potato	
	1 cup cooked brown rice	
	Total	59

Most Americans generally consume one and a half or two times their daily recommended protein allowance. In the field of nutrition, the "average adult man" is 23-50 years old, weighs 154 lbs., is 5'10" tall, and maintains a moderate activity level. The "average adult woman" is 23-50 years old, weighs 120 lbs., is 5'4" tall, and maintains a moderate activity level.

gram of fat; 4 calories per gram of protein and carbohydrates. Fats and oils are one of the main sources of calories in the American diet.

Fats come in two categories: saturated and unsaturated. Saturated, or hydrogenated, fats are hard at room temperature. Animal fats are mostly saturated, except fish fat. Unsaturated fats are liquid or soft at room temperature. The more unsaturated, the more liquid the fat. Safflower oil is the most unsaturated of fats. Vegetables fats are mostly unsaturated, except coconut oil, palm oil, and cocoa butter which are highly saturated. Coconut oil and palm oil are used by the food industry to coat crackers, cookies, food mixes, and so on, to ensure their prolonged freshness. Cocoa powder (chocolate without butter) is low in fat.

We consume fat from many sources. It is added as spreads on bread and rolls, as dressings on salads, as mayonnaise in sandwiches. A lot of fat is hidden in what we eat: occurring naturally in foods, used in commercial products, and introduced in home cooking and baking. Nuts, seeds, peanut butter, avocados, and olives are all included in the fat group. A diet to reduce cancer risk must be low in fat.

30% FAT DIET

CALORIES PER DAY	GRAMS OF FAT ALLOWED	TEASPOON EQUIVALENTS
1500	50	10
1800	60	12
2000	66	13¼
2400	80	16
3000	100	20

The 3,000 calorie, 30% fat diet allows 100 grams, or 20 teaspoons, of fat, while a typical 3,000 calorie, 42% fat American diet contains 140 grams, or 28 teaspoons, of fat.

In addition, saturated fats and cholesterol elevate the level of cholesterol in the blood. High levels of blood cholesterol lead to diseases of the heart and blood vessels. People with a high blood cholesterol level should limit saturated fat as well as total fat and cholesterol in their diet.

COUNTING THE FAT

The amount of fat you can eat will depend on the number of calories you consume. The number of calories you need depends on whether you are a woman or a man, a young active person or a sedentary middle-aged person, and so on. Generally speaking, men need more calories than women and young people more than older ones. Physical activity increases caloric needs.

To reduce a typical 3000 calorie, 42% fat American diet which contains 140 grams of fat, or 28 teaspoons, to a 30% fat one, means removing 40 grams, or 8 teaspoons, of fat. You would also drop 360 calories!

The table "30% Fat Diet" shows some examples of the actual amount of fat allowed in a 30% fat diet.

The approximate fat in some selected foods is listed in the table "Fat Content of Various Foods."

Remember, the amount of fat in your diet includes both the fat added to food and the fat which exists naturally in food. By choosing wisely and counting the amount of fat in individual foods and ingredients you use in recipes, you can control the total amount of fat in your diet. To determine calorie equivalents for fat, figure 1 teaspoon of fat equals 5 grams, and each gram of fat contains 9 calories, so 1 teaspoon of fat contains 45 calories.

Read labels on products. Fat is often listed in grams. Notice particularly the fat content of dairy products and nuts. And beware of non-dairy dairy products. They often contain high amounts of coconut or palm oil.

At the end of the day, add the total number of teaspoons of fat consumed. See how this compares with the number of teaspoons permitted for the number of calories you allow yourself.

FAT CONTENT OF VARIOUS FOODS

FOOD	AMOUNT	TOTAL FAT IN GRAMS	TOTAL FAT IN TEASPOONS*
VEGETABLES		none	none
FRUITS		none	none
except:			
Olives	5 small	4	1
Avocado	½	16	3
GRAIN PRODUCTS			
Pasta (no egg)	1 c. cooked	0.5	—
Rice			
white	1 c. cooked	0.2	—
brown	1 c. cooked	0.9	—
Breads, average	1 slice	0.6	—
French, Italian	1 slice	0.6	—
Cornbread	1 piece	3.8	¾
White	1 slice	0.7	—
Whole wheat	1 slice	0.7	—
Raisin	1 slice	0.6	—
Rye, pumpernickel	1 slice	0.3	—
Hamburger roll	1	2.2	½
Granola	½ c. commercial	8	1½
NUTS & SEEDS			
Cashews	1 oz. = 14 large	13.1	2½
Walnuts	1 oz. = 15 halves	15.1	3
Pistachio	1 oz. = 50	16.1	3¼
Almonds	1 oz. = 25	16.2	3¼
Sunflower seeds	¼ c.	16.8	3¼
Peanuts (dry-roasted)	¼ c.	17.6	3½
Filberts	1 oz. = 25	19.1	3¾
Pecans	1 oz. = 24 halves	22	4½
Macadamia nuts	1 oz. = 12	23.5	4¾

*rounded values

FOOD	AMOUNT	TOTAL FAT IN GRAMS	TOTAL FAT IN TEASPOONS
LEGUMES	1 c.	less than 1	—
MILK PRODUCTS			
Skim milk, buttermilk	1 c.	0.4	—
Frozen yogurt	½ c.	1.5	¼
Sherbet	½ c	1.9	¼
1% milk	1 c.	2.6	½
Ice milk	½ c.	2.8	½
2% milk	1 c.	5	1
Low fat yogurt	1 c.	4	1
Regular yogurt	1 c.	8	1½
Ice cream, regular	½ c.	8	1½
Whole milk	1 c.	9	1¾
Ice cream, rich	½ c.	15	3
Half & half	½ c.	16	3
Sour cream	½ c.	16	3
Whipping cream	½ c.	24	5
CHEESES			
Cottage cheese, 2%	½ c.	2.2	½
Reduced Calorie Laughing Cow	1 oz.	3	½
Mozzarella, skim	1 oz.	2	½
Lite-Line (Borden)	1 oz.	3	½
Hickory Lite-Line	1 oz.	3	½
Weight-Watcher	1 oz.	2	½
Ricotta, part skim	1 oz.	2	½
Cottage cheese, 4%	½ c.	4.2	1
Mozzarella, part skim	1 oz.	4.5	1
Light cream cheese	1 oz.	5	1
Parmesan (grated)	¼ c.	6	1¼
Mozzarella	1 oz.	6	1¼
Feta	1 oz.	6	1¼
Green River cheddar	1 oz.	7	1½
Neufchatel cream cheese	1 oz.	7	1½
Ricotta	1 oz.	4	1

FOOD	AMOUNT	TOTAL FAT IN GRAMS	TOTAL FAT IN TEASPOONS
CHEESES, continued			
Cheddar, gruyere, jack, blue, etc.	1 oz.	9-10	2
Cream cheese	1 oz.	10	2
Brie, Camembert	1 oz.	13-15	3
FISH & SHELLFISH, POULTRY, MEATS (COOKED)			
White flesh fish (cod, halibut, sole, snapper, perch, haddock, trout)	3 oz.	0-1	—
Shellfish	3 oz.	0-1	—
Tuna, packed in water	3 oz.	1	¼
Salmon, pink	3 oz.	3.2	¾
Chicken, turkey, no skin, white	3 oz.	4	1
Veal, venison	3 oz.	5	1
Tuna, canned in oil	3 oz.	8	1½
Bacon	2 strips	7.5	1½
Chicken, turkey, no skin, dark	3 oz.	8.4	1¾
Beef, flank, round, sirloin, 10% fat	3 oz.	8.5	1¾
Spareribs	3 small	10	2
Salmon, chinook	3 oz.	13.3	2⅔
Pork, lamb	3 oz.	12	2½
Ground beef, 25% fat	3 oz.	21.5	4½
LUNCHEON MEATS			
Turkey products	1 oz.	1.5	¼
Bologna	1 oz.	8	1½
Salami, dry	1 oz.	10	2
Wiener	one	13	2½
EGGS			
White	1	0.5	—
Yolk	1	5.5	1
Whole egg	1	6	1¼

FOOD	AMOUNT	TOTAL FAT IN GRAMS	TOTAL FAT IN TEASPOONS
FATS & SPREADS			
Catsup, mustard	1 Tbsp.	less than 1	—
Imitation mayonnaise	1 Tbsp.	5	1
Diet margarine	1 Tbsp.	5	1
Miracle Whip	1 Tbsp.	6.9	1¼
Soft margarine, whipped	1 Tbsp.	8	1½
Peanut butter	1 Tbsp.	8	1½
Mayonnaise	1 Tbsp.	11	2
Margarine	1 Tbsp.	12	2½
Butter	1 Tbsp.	14	3
Oils—all	1 Tbsp.	14	3
SALAD DRESSINGS			
Commercial "low-calorie," "diet"	1 Tbsp.	1	¼
French	1 Tbsp.	5.4	1
Roquefort, 1000 island	1 Tbsp.	7.6	1½
Italian	1 Tbsp.	8.4	1¾
SNACKS			
Bagel	1	less than 1	—
Popcorn, plain	1 c.	0.3	—
Pretzels	10	less than 1	—
Melba toast, matzoh	1	less than 1	—
Muffin, whole wheat	1	1.1	¼
Saltines	4	1.4	¼
Gingersnaps	4	1.2	¼
Corn chips	½ c.	6	1¼
Popcorn, buttered	1 c.	2	½
Triscuits	4	3	½
Chocolate chip cookies	2	4.4	1
Oreo cookies	2	4.5	1
Chocolate cupcake	1	5	1
Doughnut, raised	1	9.9	2
Peach crisp	1 slice	6.4	1¼

FOOD	AMOUNT	TOTAL FAT IN GRAMS	TOTAL FAT IN TEASPOONS
SNACKS, continued			
Chocolate bar	1 oz.	10	2
Croissant, plain	1	10	2
Double crust peach pie	1 slice	12	2¼
Potato chips	1 oz.	12.5	2½
FAST FOODS			
Pizza, cheese, mushroom	1 slice	4.4	1
Typical milkshake, chocolate	1	8.4	1¾
Typical hamburger	1	10	2
Typical cheeseburger	1	14	3
French fries	1 serving	14	3
Big Mac hamburger	1	33	6½

CONSUMING MORE FIBER

The typical American diet is low in fiber. It is estimated that Americans consume about 20 grams of dietary fiber per day. The American Cancer Society recommends increasing that amount by at least half, to 30 grams per day.

There is no fiber in food from animal sources. The main dietary sources of fiber are legumes, whole grains, fruits, and vegetables. These foods also are low in fat and many are good sources of vitamins A and C, so they fit well with the American Cancer Society dietary guidelines.

You can increase your fiber consumption by eating whole grain breads; using whole wheat flours, or a mixture of whole wheat and white in baking; serving brown rice, barley, bulgur, or buckwheat by themselves or combined with other foods; using dried beans or lentils in soups, salads, and stews or in dips; adding wheat or oat bran to casseroles.

BEST SOURCES OF DIETARY FIBER

Dried beans, peas, lentils

Bran cereals—All Bran, Raisin Bran, Most, Shredded Wheat

Whole wheat and whole grain products—rye, oats, buckwheat, stone ground cornmeal, barley

Sweet corn, potatoes with skin, peas

Broccoli (very high), spinach, kale, Swiss chard, carrots, Brussels sprouts, green snap beans

Raspberries, strawberries, plums, pears, apples (especially with skin), bananas, cherries

Figs, apricots, dates, raisins, prunes

Almonds, peanuts, walnuts, Brazil nuts

Although all are good sources of fiber, these foods are listed in order of fiber content. Dried beans, peas, and lentils provide the most in the group; nuts provide the least. Remember, nuts are also high in fat.

GETTING ENOUGH FIBER

FOOD	GRAMS*
2 slices whole wheat bread	5
1 cup cooked brown rice or bulgur, or 1 small baked potato with skin	5
¾ cup whole grain cereal	5
1 piece fruit	5
1 cup cooked vegetables	5
⅓ cup cooked beans, peas, lentils	5
Total	30

*Average values.

This is an example of how 30 grams of fiber can be obtained in a single day. With some practice, you can achieve a 30-gram-a-day fiber intake.

You can also choose high fiber commercial cereals (Shredded Wheat, Oat Bran, Natural All Bran); add bran to dry or cooked cereals; eat air-popped popcorn (unbuttered) as a snack; add red beans, peas, or garbanzos to vegetable salads; eat more fresh fruit, especially apples, pears, peaches, and oranges; eat more fresh vegetables, especially broccoli, carrots, and peas.

The table "Getting Enough Fiber" shows how you might reach a dietary intake of 30 grams of fiber in one day. The table "Amounts of Foods Containing 5 Grams of Fiber" shows how some foods compare in the amount of dietary fiber they contain.

AMOUNTS OF FOODS CONTAINING 5 GRAMS OF FIBER

FOOD	AMOUNT
Whole wheat bread	2 slices
White bread	6½ slices
Brown rice	1¾ cups
White rice	4 cups
Shredded wheat cereal	1⅓ cups
Cheerios-type cereal	6 cups
Raw bran	3 Tbsp.
Cooked beans, peas lentils	⅓ cup
Lettuce salad	5 cups
Celery, diced	2½ cups
Strawberries, raspberries	⅔ cup
Oranges	2 medium

Dietary fiber is made of different substances which all have a role to play in the maintenance of our health. It is best to choose fiber from ALL sources.

VITAMINS A & C

The American Cancer Society dietary guidelines include a recommendation to consume foods rich in vitamins A and C on a daily basis. Eating 2 or 3 servings of vegetables and 3 or 4 pieces of fruit is considered appropriate in a prudent cancer prevention diet. You will notice that the vegetables of the mustard family recommended by the Society are also in the following lists.

BEST LOW FAT SOURCES OF BETA CAROTENE AND VITAMIN A

DARK GREEN & DEEP YELLOW VEGETABLES

Beet greens, cooked
Broccoli
Carrots
Chard, cooked
Chicory, cooked
Collard greens, cooked
Dandelion greens, cooked
Kale, cooked
Mustard greens, cooked

Parsley
Pumpkin
Spinach
Sweet potatoes
Tomatoes
Tomato juice
Turnip greens, cooked
Watercress
Winter squash

DEEP YELLOW & RED FRUITS

Apricots, canned
Apricots, dried
Apricots, fresh
Cantaloupe
Mango

Nectarine
Papaya
Persimmon
Plantain
Watermelon

All other vegetables and fruits contain Vitamin A. They may not be as rich in this nutrient as those listed but are nonetheless excellent food in a diet to reduce cancer risk.

BEST SOURCES OF VITAMIN C

VEGETABLES

Broccoli
Collard greens, cooked
Kale, cooked
Parsley

Peppers, green—hot chili, sweet
Tomatoes/tomato juice
Turnip greens, cooked

FRUITS

Cantaloupe
Grapefruit/grapefruit juice
Guava
Kiwi
Lemon/lemon juice

Orange/orange juice
Papaya
Strawberries
Tangerine
Watermelon

All other vegetables and fruits contain Vitamin C. They may not be as rich in this nutrient as those listed but are nonetheless excellent food to include in a diet to reduce cancer risk.

ADDING IT ALL UP

In practical terms, a cancer prevention eating style means:

- Eating more foods from the vegetable world (grains, legumes, fruit, and vegetables);

- Eating fewer foods from the animal world and choosing the low fat varieties (low fat dairy products including low fat cheeses, fish and shellfish, poultry, rabbit, venison, and lean cuts of veal, pork, lamb, and beef);

- Limiting the consumption of high fat meats, whole milk dairy products (including butter, cheeses, and cream), avocados, olives, nuts, chocolate, coconut oil, and palm oil;

- Decreasing consumption of both added and hidden fats mentioned earlier, using less fat in recipes prepared at home, avoiding foods canned in oil and paying attention to foods eaten out; and

- Avoiding fried foods and meats and fish which are salt-cured, pickled, or smoked.

SHOPPING FOR FOODS

Reducing fat and increasing fiber in your daily diet starts at the grocery store. Under the pressure of customers, the food industry is including a list of ingredients with dietary information on a greater number of product packages than in the past. Notice the amount of fat—both saturated and unsaturated—in each product you consider buying. Remember, the ingredients are listed in the order of their amounts. A large number of products show fat, salt, or sugar as their first—and most important—ingredient. Compare products. For example, regular mayonnaise contains 11 grams of fat per tablespoon while imitation mayonnaise contains 5 grams per tablespoon.

If there is a government "standard of identity" specifying the contents of a food product, a reduced calorie version of this food must be called "imitation." It means that any serving of the food contains less fat (and fewer calories) than the original product—not that it is a fake food.

There is no official definition of food labelled "light." Read the label carefully to be sure that the product is indeed lower in fat.

A food labeled "low calories" is, in practical terms, lower in fat. The Food and Drug Administration requires that such a food contain no more than 40 calories per serving or per 100 grams (3½ ounces). Low calorie salad dressings fall into this category.

To be labeled "reduced calories" a food must be at least one-third lower in calorie content than the comparable food which has not been reduced. Foods so labeled generally are lower in fat.

Both low calorie and reduced calorie labels must list the nutritional content of the food. Choose accordingly.

The following tips and tables are to help you shop for and use foods with an eye to fat content.

Dairy Products

It is important to know that when the butterfat is reduced or removed from dairy products, only fat and cholesterol content become low or negligible while the other nutrient levels do not decrease. As a matter of fact, the calcium content of skim milk products increases. Skim milk products are simply more healthful. (See the section called About Calcium; also see Milk Products and Cheeses in the table "Fat Content of Various Foods.")

Cheeses vary greatly in amount of fat (and in cholesterol). Their fat content ranges from as low as 1% to a high of 70%. The fat content is frequently indicated on the labels and is usually expressed as grams of fat per ounce.

Low fat cheeses contain 3 grams of fat or less per ounce. They can be used as snacks or in cooking instead of medium or high fat cheeses. Medium fat cheeses contain 4-7 grams of fat per ounce. It is better to use them at meal time as a replacement for meat (1 ounce cheese = 2 ounces meat) or in cooking instead of high fat cheeses. High fat cheeses contain 8 grams of fat or more per ounce. They are to be used sparingly, if at all, as a replacement for meat (1 ounce cheese = 3 ounces meat). Buy small amounts only.

Poultry, Fish, Shellfish, Eggs, Meats

As already mentioned, fish, shellfish, and poultry are better choices than meats because they contain less fat (and fewer calories). Limit meat and poultry to 3 or 4 ounces cooked per day, fish and shellfish to 6 ounces, eggs to 1-2 per week. Dry beans, peas, lentils, garbanzos, and grains are good replacements for meat dishes. Shop accordingly.

Many fish and meat products are sold salt-cured, pickled, smoked, or canned in oil or brine. Leave them on the grocery shelf. Luncheon meats are particularly high in fat: buy the new turkey and chicken products now available.

SELECTING MILK PRODUCTS

TYPE	CHOOSE	USE LESS OFTEN
For drinking and cooking	1% milk, skim milk, evaporated skim milk, low fat dry milk buttermilk	Whole milk, 2% milk, buttermilk made from whole milk, evaporated whole milk
	Cocoa drinks, instant breakfasts	Chocolate milk
	Plain low fat yogurt. In cooking add 1 tablespoon flour or cornstarch to avoid curdling	Sour cream
Creamers	Mocha Mix, Poly-rich, powdered skim milk	Non-dairy coffee creamers,* half & half
Toppings	Sweetened plain or vanilla low fat yogurt, whipped low fat cottage cheese	Sour cream, whipping cream, non-dairy whipped toppings,* Cool Whip, IMO, Dream Whip
Frozen desserts	Ice milk, sherbet, frozen low fat yogurt, sorbet, ices, Weight-Watchers ice cream	Ice cream, Mellorine, Tofutti†
Commercial milk-based products	Gelatin-based, dry pudding mixes (add low fat milk)	Custards, puddings made with cream or whole milk or chocolate

*Beware of imitation dairy products. They often contain large amounts of coconut or palm oil, both highly saturated fats. These products are advertised as being low in cholesterol, which is true, but they are still very high in fat and are no better than the products they are meant to replace.

†Tofutti is a new frozen dessert made with tofu, skim milk, and unsaturated vegetable oils. It contains no cholesterol and little saturated fat, but it remains rather high in fat.

SELECTING CHEESES

Low Fat Cheeses

KIND OR BRAND	USE
Dry curd or 2% cottage cheese	As a snack, topping (whipped) on baked potatoes, in Mexican dishes
Skim milk farmers cheese	As a snack
Reduced Calorie Laughing Cow	Excellent as snack, spread on breads or crackers
Part-skim ricotta, Imitation mozzarella	Excellent for cooking, on pizza
Lite-Line, Lite'n Lively, Weight Watchers slices	As snacks, in cooking
Light Kraft cream cheese	Instead of Philadephia cream cheese

Medium Fat Cheeses

KIND OR BRAND	USE
4% Cottage cheese	In cooking mixed with other cheeses
Green River part-skim cheddar, Low fat cheddar, Heidi Ann	In cooking instead of whole milk cheddar
Part-skim mozzarella, ricotta, Pizza-Pal	In cooking (lasagna, pizza, manicotti, etc.)
Cheezola	For Velveeta lovers
Neufchatel	Instead of Philadelphia cream cheese
Sapsago	Instead of Parmesan

High Fat Cheeses

KIND	USE
American	Sparingly in cooking,
Blue	as spreads, or in
Brie	sandwiches
Camembert	
Cheddar	
Colby	
Cream cheese	
Feta	
Gouda	
Gruyere	
Havarti	
Jarlsberg	
Min-Chol†	
Monterey jack	
Parmesan‡	
Processed American	
Port Salut**	
Romano	
Roquefort	
Swiss	

†Min-Chol is made of skim milk and soybean oil instead of butterfat.

‡Parmesan is high in fat but is so dry, light, and pungent that it can be used in cooking (but no more than 1 tablespoon per serving).

**Port Salut is made from partially skim milk and is the lowest in fat of the high fat cheeses.

SELECTING ANIMAL PROTEIN FOODS

CHOOSE	USE LESS OFTEN
Most fish and shellfish	Smelt, caviar
Tuna canned in water	Tuna canned in oil
Rabbit, chicken, turkey, veal roast, venison	Goose, duck, veal chops
Lean ham (93% fat free)	Country ham, deviled ham
Canadian bacon	Bacon
Turkey and chicken luncheon meats	Sausages, salami, bologna, wieners, pastrami
—	Smoked meats, poultry, fish
—	Canned meats, corned beef
Round steak, rump roast, flank steak, sirloin tip	Beef, rib steak
Pot roast, stew meat	Beef, rib roast, standing rib
Ground chicken or ground turkey	Ground beef
Ground round (10-15% fat)	Hamburger (20-30% fat)
"Good" or "Standard"	"Choice" or "Prime"
Lamb leg	Most lamb cuts
—	Ground lamb
Pork sirloin, roast	Pork ribs, spareribs
Tongue	Organ meats

The items to use less often are all high in fat. Remember that any meats which are salt-cured, nitrite-cured, or smoked have carcinogen-containing tars, so should be eaten sparingly.

While eggs and organ meats do not contain a large amount of fat they do contain high amounts of cholesterol. People with high blood cholesterol should limit their intake of these foods.

Fats and Oils

These are the foods to watch for most carefully. Saturated, unsaturated, solid, liquid, of animal orgin, of vegetable origin, added or hidden—all fats are to be decreased in a cancer prevention diet. Read labels. More about fats and oils can be found in the section called Cooking & Baking.

Although it is always preferable to eat homemade food because the amounts of fat used can be controlled, this is not always feasible. Here is a list of high fat commercial products and suitable replacements.

SELECTING COMMERCIAL PRODUCTS

CHOOSE	USE LESS OFTEN
Hard candies, jelly beans, marshmallows, meringues	Chocolate candies, caramels
Fig bars, graham crackers, ginger snaps, vanilla wafers	Cookies, high fat
Fruit desserts, open fruit tarts	Pies, double crust
Muffins	Pastries, doughnuts, croissants
Homemade low fat cakes, angel food cake, puddings made with commercial puddings to mix with skim milk	Rich cakes
Bagels, pita bread, English muffins, French bread, Italian	Specialty breads
Pretzels, unbuttered popcorn, plain saltines, Scandinavian flat breads, rice cakes, Bremner crackers	High fat crackers
Corn or whole wheat tortilla	Flour tortilla
Baked potatoes	French fried potatoes, fresh or frozen
Granola without coconut and nuts	Standard granola or granola bars
Plain frozen foods	Canned or creamed frozen foods
Vegetarian canned beans	Canned pork and beans
Lean Cuisine-type frozen entrees	Standard frozen entrees
Vegetarian, Canadian bacon pizza	Sausage, pepperoni pizza

ABOUT CALCIUM

In recent years, researchers have probed deeper into the role of calcium in the formation and the maintenance of bone health. They have found

SOURCES OF CALCIUM

FOOD	AMOUNT	MG. PER SERVING
Yogurt, plain low fat	1 cup	415
Yogurt, fruit flavored low fat	1 cup	345
Milk, skim or low fat	1 cup	300
Buttermilk	1 cup	300
Nonfat dry milk	4 Tbsp.	200
Part-skim mozzarella cheese	1 ounce	200
Collard/mustard greens	½ cup, cooked	175
Buttermilk pancakes	3 (4-inch)	175
Salmon, canned	3 ounces	165
Cottage cheese, low fat	1 cup	150
Tofu	3½ ounces	130
Shrimp, canned	3 ounces	100
Garbanzo beans	½ cup, cooked	75
Okra, broccoli	½ cup, cooked	70
Soybeans	½ cup, cooked	70
Orange	1 medium	60
Dark molasses	1 Tbsp.	60
Lettuce	1 cup	60
Corn tortilla	1, 6″ each	60
Clams	½ cup	55
Rutabaga, green beans, cabbage, bean sprouts, pinto, kidney beans	½ cup	50
Muffin, corn bread	1 average	50
Bread, whole wheat	2 slices	50
Egg substitutes	¼ cup	30
Berries, pineapple	½ cup	10

that the need for calcium increases as we grow older. There is also increasing concern that the American diet does not contain enough calcium. This is especially true for women. The maintenance of bone health—the avoidance of osteoporosis, or "brittle bones"—is a complex matter involving many factors, but the need for a good supply of calcium from the diet is evident.

The National Academy of Science's Recommended Daily Allowance (RDA) for calcium is 800 milligrams per person. Some scientists recommend higher intakes for women—1000 to 1500 milligrams per day—particularly because the American diet is high in protein and the higher the protein level in the diet, the higher the need for calcium.

Many people are concerned that following a diet low in fat means consuming fewer dairy products and, as a result, being deficient in calcium. This need not be a concern. First of all, a diet low in fat does not mean one with few dairy products. There are plenty of low fat dairy products (low fat milks, yogurts, cheeses, ice milk, and so on). These products contain as much as and sometimes more calcium than whole milk products. Secondly, there are other good sources of calcium in the world of food. The table "Sources of Calcium" will help you choose good low fat sources of calcium.

COOKING & BAKING

Here are some pointers for preparing food so that it has the least amount of fat possible and the most nutritional value.

Vegetables

Serve them raw, marinated in vinegar or lemon juice and herbs. Frozen vegetables can also be used. If you are cooking vegetables, steaming them will help keep their color, taste, and nutrients. If you wish to boil them, do so in a minimum of water. Vegetables can be sautéed or stir-fried quickly in a minimum of fat, without fat in a nonstick frying pan, in a pan using nonstick spray, or cooked without fat in a microwave oven.

Poultry and Meats

Proper cooking of poultry and meats is not complicated:

- Trim all visible fat from poultry and meats, and skin poultry to remove the layer of fat underneath.

- Stretch a small amount of poultry or meat in casseroles and stews by stir-frying. The meat will be a spice for the vegetables and grains.

- Roast in an uncovered cooking pot in the oven. Place poultry or meat on a rack in the roasting pan: the fat will drip off during cooking. Cook at low temperatures: more fat will drip off.

- Stew on top of the stove or bake in a covered pan with added liquid —broth, wine, or water. Less tender, low fat cuts of meat retain their moisture better this way.

- Sauté or Stir-fry, the French or the Chinese way. These methods allow the food to be cooked quickly in the minimum of fat. Cut poultry, meat, or fish in very small pieces to facilitate quick cooking. Try sautéing without fat in a nonstick frying pan or with a nonstick spray on the pan.

- Broiling is not recommended. A possible link between broiling and mutagen formation is being studied.

- NEVER fry poultry or meat. The same caution applies as for broiling. Also, frying requires additional fat: a healthful diet reduces fat.

Gravies, Stocks, and Broths

Stocks and broths for gravies are best prepared ahead of time. When meat or poultry are cooked, pour juices in a container. Chill in refrigerator; the fat will harden and rise to the top of the container. Discard the solidified fat and use the dark, fragrant juice underneath to make gravy in your own favorite way. Juices can be stored in the freezer for later use. Commercial canned beef broth although high in salt is usually relatively low in fat and can be used in low fat cookery. Open the can after chilling in the refrigerator and remove any visible fat. Thicken sauces with cornstarch which, unlike flour, does not require mixing with fat.

A fine chicken broth is easily made at home. Look under Chicken Broth, Quick in the Index. Like commercial beef broth, commercial chicken broth is usually relatively low in fat and can be used in low fat cookery. As with beef broth, chill the the can first, then open it and remove any visible fat.

Fish

Fish is the supreme convenience food. It cooks quickly, and fish steaks can be cooked from the frozen state, unlike other steaks. Be careful not to overcook fish: it can become tough or fall apart.

Many people not familiar with the delicate flavor of most fish may want to add some herbs or spices. The following work well with fish: lemon, lemon juice, dill weed, fennel seeds, garlic, onion, sweet basil, paprika, saffron, parsley, thyme, curry powder.

These are the basic rules for cooking fish:

- Cook 10 minutes per 1 inch of thickness (measure thickest part with a ruler) or until opaque and flaky. Double cooking time for frozen fish.

- Bake with onion, tomatoes, wine or fish broth to keep fish moist and flavorful. Bake in 350° oven until flaky.

- Poach in water, skim milk, or wine, barely covering a single layer of fish in a pan. Season, bring to a boil, cover and simmer for 10 minutes. Remove delicately.

- Steam on a steaming rack 1 to 2 inches from simmering liquid in a deep cooking pot. Cover tightly, reduce heat, and steam until flaky. Seafood is excellent prepared this way.

- Sauté in a small amount of vegetable oil or stir fry with vegetables and serve over rice.

- Cook in a microwave oven, without fat, about 3 minutes per pound.

- Broiling is not recommended. A possible link between broiling and mutagen formation is being studied.

- NEVER fry fish. The same caution applies as for broiling. Also, frying requires additional fat: a healthful diet reduces fat.

Eggs

Eggs can be poached, hard or soft boiled, or scrambled in a nonstick frying pan. Just as with meat, poultry, and fish, never fry eggs. (Also see the section called About the Recipes.)

Fats and Oils

The recipes in this book already have a reduced fat content. Use the table "Fat Content of Various Foods" to help determine the amount of fat in recipes you find elsewhere and recipes already collected. The tables "Selecting Milk Products," "Selecting Cheeses," and "Selecting Animal Protein Foods" will be useful in finding alternatives for various ingredients. The following recommendation tables will also help reduce the fat content of foods you prepare.

Hidden fats are present naturally in certain foods. We cannot say often enough that these foods should be consumed sparingly and/or substitutes used where possible.

The table of substitutions is provided for quick reference when preparing recipes. After making substitutions in a recipe you may find a need to change the amounts slightly to make a totally satisfying dish.

REDUCING ADDED FATS

IN SPREADS

Butter and margarine:
  Omit on rolls, pancakes, waffles or, if absolutely necessary, replace with: jam, jelly, syrup, honey. Choose a delicious, crusty bread which does not need any improvement—delete the spread.

Butter, margarine, sour cream, or IMO
   Omit on baked potatoes and replace with whipped cottage cheese
   or plain low fat yogurt with chives or Mock Sour Cream (see Index).
Mayonnaise or peanut butter:
   Omit on sandwiches and replace with mustard or cranberry sauce on
   turkey and chicken; imitation mayonnaise on tuna. Do not use both
   margarine and mayonnaise or margarine and peanut butter. Use
   more jelly than peanut butter on peanut butter and jelly sandwiches.

IN SALAD DRESSINGS

High fat salad dressings (Blue Cheese, 1000 Island, Miracle Whip,
Italian, sour cream base)
   Use less or use lemon juice with herbs, low calorie commercial salad
   dressings, ranch mixes with buttermilk and yogurt, French dressing.

IN TOPPINGS

Flavored commercial toppings, sour cream, Cool Whip:
   Omit or use whipped low fat cottage cheese, low fat plain or vanilla
   yogurt, Mock Sour Cream (see Index), or powdered sugar.

IN COOKING

Butter lard, margarine, and oils
   Cut amount in half or use nonstick pans to sauté, boil, or poach
   food, or cook in microwave with no added fat.

IN BAKING

Margarine, butter, shortening
   Cut down amount of fat indicated in recipe to no more than
   2 tablespoons per serving. To thicken sauces, use cornstarch in place
   of flour; cornstarch will mix well without adding fat. Substitute
   ¾ tablespoon oil or soft margarine for 1 tablespoon hard margarine
   or butter.

REDUCING HIDDEN FATS

Meats and Cheeses
   See best choices in tables, "Selecting Animal Protein Foods" and
   "Selecting Cheeses." Also see About the Recipes.
Nuts
   These are about 50% fat. Use sparingly as snacks. In cooking use no
   more than 1-2 teaspoons per serving.
Avocado, olives
   Use sparingly.
Chocolate, carob
   Replace with cocoa powder

SUBSTITUTIONS

IN PLACE OF	USE
1 tablespoon margarine/butter	¾ tablespoon oil or soft diet margarine
1 whole egg	2 egg whites, or commercial egg substitute according to package directions
2 whole eggs	2 egg whites + 1 whole egg or equivalent egg substitute
1 cup whole milk	1 cup skim milk
1 cup sour cream	1 cup plain low fat yogurt + ¼ cup imitation mayonnaise or use Mock Sour Cream (see Index)
1 ounce square of chocolate	3 tablespoons cocoa powder + 1 teaspoon vegetable oil

HOMEMADE EGG SUBSTITUTE

6 egg whites
¼ cup nonfat powdered milk
1 tablespoon vegetable oil

Combine all ingredients in a mixing bowl and blend until smooth.
Store in jar in refrigerator up to 1 week. Also freezes well. Can be used
the same as commercial egg substitutes in baking and is considerably
cheaper! To prepare as scrambled eggs: cook slowly over low heat in a
nonstick fry pan. Makes 1 cup.

SNACKING

From a nutritional point of view, there is nothing wrong with snacking.
Because low fat, high fiber foods are filling without contributing many
calories to the diet there is room for extra food during the course of the
day. Well chosen, snacks can complement a well-balanced diet.

If you have read this book this far, and consulted the tables listing the
fat content of foods as well as the tips about shopping for and using low
fat food products, you have a reasonable idea of what constitutes a
healthful snack: one that is low in fat, low in calories, and high in fiber.
Good nutrition suggests that it should also be low in salt and sugar. To
further help you choose healthful snacks, here are some tips.

Fruits

All fresh fruits are good, except avocados and olives, which are high in
fat. Fruit canned in water or light syrup is also acceptable, as are frozen
fruits. Fruit ices (including sorbets) and sherbets are excellent.

Vegetables

All fresh, frozen, and canned vegetables make excellent snacks. Carrot
and celery sticks are fine, but try cauliflower, zucchini, turnips, and other

vegetables. For a fancier snack, marinate vegetables in lemon juice, vinegar, and herbs or in low calorie commercial salad dressing.

Breads

There are so many kinds: bagels, cornbread, crumpets, English muffins, French, Italian, pita (pocket), rye, sourdough, whole wheat, multigrain, corn or whole wheat tortillas. Use them with fruit butters, low fat dips or reduced calorie cheeses.

Cereals

All-Bran, Cheerios, Cornflakes, Grape-Nuts, Puffed Rice, Raisin Bran, Rice Krispies, and Shredded Wheat are some of the cereals you can snack on, using low fat milk. Air-popped popcorn is an excellent snack; season popcorn with pepper, herbs, or a little Parmesan cheese.

Crackers

There are low fat crackers on the market: Ak-Mak, Bremner, Cracottes, matzoh, Melba Toast, unsalted pretzels, rice cakes, Ry-Krisp, Scandinavian flat breads, unsalted soda crackers. Use them in the same way you would breads.

Dairy Products

Use low fat milk or buttermilk, low fat cheese, low fat yogurt (add your own fruit), ices, sherbet, or ice milk.

Baked Goods

The best baked snacks are those made at home with low fat ingredients. Muffins can be a snack as well as a breakfast or dinner food. Of the commercial products, fig bars, ginger snaps, vanilla wafers, and graham crackers are among the lowest in fat.

Beverages

There is a lot to be said for water, with or without lemon juice or lemon peel. Buttermilk and other low fat milks are good. Homemade milkshakes can be made with low fat ingredients: sherbet, cocoa powder, fruit, and low fat milk. Fruit juices are acceptable, although fresh fruits which are higher in fiber and lower in calories are preferable. On a cold day, cocoa made with low fat milk and cocoa powder or commercial instant breakfast can be a treat as well as nourishing.

This and That

Leftover soup or salad can make a delicious snack. When a more substantial snack is wanted, also consider beans. Refried beans and a corn tortilla make a good burrito. Hummus makes a nice filling for pocket bread.

About Other Snacking Foods

Peanut butter, nuts, and seeds are nutritious, but high in fat (50% on the average)—too high to be eaten as snacks unless the rest of the diet is very low in fat.

Commercial granola bars and granolas are high in fat (usually coconut oil), sugar, and calories. Again, possible additions to a diet, but only if you can afford the calories and the fat.

Health snacks and candies are often fine, but read the labels: some are very high in fat, coconut or coconut oil, and sugar. Wheat germ also contains fat. Corn chips, soy chips, and banana chips are fried in fat.

Regular soft drinks are high in sugar; diet pop is high in sodium.

EATING OUT

Many Americans eat at least one of every three meals out. It is possible to follow a nutritious diet, one low in fat and high in fiber, while eating away from home, but it requires some planning.

First of all, remember that it is your decision to follow a prudent diet. Your health is important enough to you that you are committed to some specific food choices and you want them to be a permanent part of your life.

In a restaurant, study the menu. Establish a good rapport with your server; ask how the food is prepared. Make specific requests. Ask that butter not be used in the preparation of your food; if a fat is necessary, ask that vegetable oil or margarine be used. Choose simply prepared entrées at dinner. Request that fish, shellfish, poultry, or lean meat be poached, steamed, or baked. Ask for lemon slices, chopped parsley, or green onions to enhance your entrée. If you order an entrée with sauce, ask for the sauce to be served on the side. Wine sauces are lighter in fat —Bordelaise, for example. If the serving size is too large, ask your server to package some portion to be taken home.

The world is changing: the food industry and the restaurant industry are aware that an increasing number of their customers want and need more healthful choices. Many restaurants now offer dishes which conform to the guidelines of the American Heart Association. Ask for these dishes. They will be similar to those which follow the American Cancer Society guidelines.

At a friend's house, discreetly but firmly tell your host or hostess— in advance, preferably—that you are eating differently now for health reasons. Everyone defers to the needs of a person with diabetes who must take the illness into consideration when choosing foods. You, too, have a need: to prevent illness. If the speaking out approach does not fit you, just pass the sauce, the butter, or the rolls; take small portions of high fat foods.

If you travel by air, contact the airline 24 hours before you leave. Airlines offer a choice of low fat, vegetarian, or low cholesterol menus on request. Ask for details about the food served from these menus. Assert your right to choose.

BEST EATING OUT CHOICES

These suggestions are for those who want to follow a strict diet or who eat out too often for those meals to be viewed as special occasions.

For breakfast

- Cereal, cooked or unsweetened dry, with low fat milk
- Fruit, with or without low fat cottage cheese

- Waffles or pancakes with syrup and without butter or margarine
- Bread, toast, or English muffins with fruit butters, jams, or jellies

For lunch

- Shrimp or crab cocktail with hot sauce
- Soup—minestrone, lentil, split pea, or clear
- Salad, especially one you can make yourself at a salad bar.
- Omit bacon, egg, and cheese on salads and choose vinaigrette, French, Italian, or ranch dressing
- Fruit salad
- Turkey, chicken, or tuna sandwich without mayonnaise
- Small hamburger without mayonnaise
- Pasta with marinara sauce or salsa sauce
- Baked potato with low fat cottage cheese and chives
- Pizza with mushrooms, tomato, shrimp or Canadian bacon
- Vegetarian chili, enchilada, or bean burrito—hold the cheese and sour cream

For dinner

- Appetizers

Vegetables—fresh or marinated in vinegar, soups (see lunch choices), salads with vinaigrette dressing, fruit (cantaloupe, grapefruit, etc.)

- Entrées

Fish, shellfish, poultry, or lean meat prepared with little or no fat— baked, poached, steamed, sautéed, roasted, stir-fried—or pasta with a vegetable sauce topping

- Side Dishes

Vegetables and starches (a good size side dish can be eaten as an entrée; select dishes with no cheese and not au gratin or scalloped)

- Breads

If the rest of the meal is low in fat you may want or need extra calories —such as a crusty bread

- Desserts

Fresh, baked, or poached fruit, fruit compote, sherbet, sorbet, ice, fruit meringue, angel food cake, simple fruit tart

- Beverages

Fresh or sparkling water with lemon or lime, wine with sparkling water, cocktail mixed with sparkling water or soda

If you have in mind foods that are not listed in the best eating out choices, check the fat content before you go out to eat. Some foods are clearly undesirable in a healthful diet low in fat. Here are some of the foods to pass up: bacon, sausage, eggs, sweet rolls, pastries, croissants, whole milk, cream, whole milk cheese, quiche, cold cuts, foods made with mayonnaise such as potato salad and coleslaw, all fried foods.

Remember, vegetables and starches (grains, pasta, potatoes) are the mainstay of an eating style that minimizes fat. Eat plenty of them but make certain they are steamed, boiled, or baked and served without butter or sauces.

Brownbagging

Lunch is a common meal eaten out. If you are at work and brown-bagging it, many of the best eating out choices listed for lunch can be good choices. Use a wide mouth thermos to carry hot, low fat leftovers from the day before—soups, casseroles, stews—or cold salads. Complete the lunch with some fruit and bread.

Fast Foods

You may only have time for a quick lunch. You do not have to eat the standard fast food fare: burger, French fries, soda or shake. Many fast food restaurants are responding to customer demand for vegetables, fruit, wholesome breads. Look for a fast food restaurant with a salad bar. Often you will find beans to add protein to your salad. Another good choice is a baked potato with a vegetable or low fat yogurt topping, followed by fresh fruit. Many more places are serving fresh fruit. Fruit with low fat yogurt topping plus a roll makes a nutritious lunch. Beware of the fish and poultry choices. They are breaded and fried and higher in fat than a hamburger. Finally, if choices are limited, a plain, small hamburger is acceptable.

Frozen Dinners and Entrées

You want to be able to make a quick evening meal sometimes. A variety of frozen foods claim to be light, gourmet, or calorie-conscious. Laboratory-tested dinners, including Lean Cuisine, Weight Watchers, Le Menu, Dinner Classics, Gorton's, and Mrs. Paul's, have been found to be good sources of protein and B vitamins, and fair sources of iron. Although some of the new frozen dinners and entrées are lower in calories than the standard dinners, many are still high in fat content.

Steakhouses

These restaurants might be considered for a special occasion. However, the steaks are likely to be Prime or Choice—the highest in fat of meat grades. Most steak servings will be large; ask for the portion size you want. Chicken is usually fried. Salads tend to be heavily dressed, so ask for a vinaigrette-style dressing on the side. If you have a baked potato ask for it to be served without butter, sour cream, or bacon and with chives.

Ethnic Foods

For a different taste, eat at a restaurant offering ethnic foods. Many ethnic restaurants serve dishes prepared with little fat.

Chinese and Indochinese. Grains and vegetables are more prominent than animal protein foods in Chinese and Indochinese cooking. Many dishes are prepared by boiling, steaming, sautéing, or stir-frying in vegetable oil. Avoid fried choices. Dry noodles have been deep fried so are high in fat. Szechuan-style food is high in fat when the meat is first fried in hot oil. To limit salt ask that soy sauce only be served on the side. Thai and Vietnamese cooking is very low in fat and high in taste.

Far Eastern. The Far Eastern restaurants, with their preference for yogurt in the making of sauces for vegetables, lentils, garbanzo beans, and grains, are recommended. Recipes are high in spices. It is best to avoid lamb dishes: they can be high in fat.

French. You can enjoy a French restaurant if you choose wine sauces over richer sauces and choose simple entrées of the provinces, such as bouillabaisse or coq au vin. Stay away from the au gratin dishes, which often come with toppings not only of cheese but butter. The French make many simple vegetable dishes and fat-free desserts such as pears in wine and sorbets.

Greek. While many appetizers and entrées are made with lamb or phyllo dough, both high in fat, such appetizers as tzatziki, made with yogurt (preferably low fat) and cucumbers, and entrées such as plaki, fish cooked with tomatoes, onions, and garlic, are excellent. Have your entrée with rice or pita bread. Greek salads can be high in fat. Request that olives and feta cheese be removed before serving.

Italian. It is true that many Italian dishes include pasta. In an eating style low in fat, pasta is a good choice—so long as the dish is not filled with fatty meat or cheese, or served with butter or cream sauce. White or red clam sauce is fine, as are marsala sauce and tomato-based marinara without meat. Pasta primavera offers fresh vegetables. Chicken, shellfish, and fish dishes simply prepared are also options. Heavy crust pizzas with mushrooms, tomato, Canadian bacon or shrimp are fine. Italian ices make a refreshing dessert.

Japanese. Fish plays a prominent part in Japanese cooking. Just remember to bypass deep-fried dishes like tempura. Look for tofu (soybean curd) dishes which are protein-rich while low in fat. You will find a variety of dishes prepared with a minimum of fat. The steamed rice is a good source of carbohydrate. To limit salt, ask that it be used sparingly.

Mexican. Whole grains have a prominent place in Mexican dishes. Choose corn not flour tortillas, and make sure they have been baked, not fried. A shrimp or chicken tostada served on a corn tortilla is a good choice. Request that sour cream, cheese, and avocado not be included. Rice and beans with tomatoes, onions, and spices are wholesome—if the beans are not prepared with lard.

Middle Eastern. You will find vegetables, grains, and spices in abundance. Try couscous (steamed, finely cracked wheat) topped with vegetables or chicken. Avoid dishes made with phyllo dough or cheese. Lamb dishes can be high in fat and some involve broiling. Fresh fruit—grapes and melons especially—is often served for dessert.

Health Food/Vegetarian. Changing eating habits have resulted in more restaurants which serve a variety of salads, dishes with beans and grains, yogurt-based foods, and whole grain breads. Some dishes are likely to be high in fat because they are prepared with a large quantity of oil, high fat dairy products, or nuts and seeds. Ask if eggs or whole milk products have been used. If your meal has been low in fat, fruit bread makes a sweet ending.

As you can see, eating out can be healthful as well as pleasurable. If you wish to strictly follow the American Cancer Society dietary guidelines, you can, and still enjoy a delicious meal. Remember, though, there is no reason why, on a special occasion, you should forego a meal that does not meet the guidelines or the general rules for good health. Balance such a meal with very low fat meals the day before—and enjoy yourself with a clear conscience.

ABOUT THE RECIPES

In this book, the focus is rightly on the the American Cancer Society Interim Dietary Guidelines. Information is given on how to best implement them while maintaining a balanced diet. The recipes have been reviewed to ensure that they conform to the guidelines. The Society also shares the concern of dietitians for overall good nutrition. Here are some comments about other elements in food: cholesterol, salt, and sugars, and how they were treated in the recipes in addition to fats and fiber.

Cholesterol

While the evidence of a relationship between high dietary cholesterol and the incidence of cancer remains inconclusive, a National Institutes of Health-sponsored Cholesterol Consensus conference in 1984 clearly established that most Americans have blood cholesterol levels undesirably high because of a high cholesterol (and fat, and saturated fat) intake. Elevated blood cholesterol levels are a major risk factor in the development of heart and blood vessel diseases. For cholesterol we have adopted a prudent approach and followed the 1985 recommendations, *Dietary Guidelines for Americans*, of the U.S. Department of Health and Human Services, decreasing the cholesterol content of our recipes. We have:

- Reduced the number of eggs in recipes or replaced 1 whole egg with 2 egg whites or the equivalent in homemade or commercial egg substitutes (the cholesterol is only in the egg yolk)

- Replaced butter or animal fat with margarines or vegetable oils (which contain no natural cholesterol)

- Replaced whole milk with skim milk or low fat milk to reduce the amount of cholesterol along with the fat

- Replaced high fat cheeses with part skim ones and reduced the amounts commonly used (about 1/4 cup low fat cheese for 4 servings in a main dish or 8 servings in a side dish)

- Replaced sour or whipping cream with plain low fat yogurt or whipped low fat cottage cheese

- Limited the portions of lean meats or poultry to 3-4 ounces per serving, and fish and shellfish to 6 ounces (despite having cholesterol amounts similar to other meats, fish is preferable because of its low unsaturated fat content and because of some specific long chain fatty acids—omega 3 type—which help lower the blood cholesterol levels. Hence the more liberal recommended amounts).

- Excluded any organ meats (gizzard, liver, heart, etc.) in the recipes as they are extremely high in cholesterol.

Salt (*Sodium*)

There is at the moment no evidence linking salt, or the sodium element in salt, and cancer. However, high blood pressure is common in this country and a reduction of salt in the diet helps lower it. Besides, too high a salt intake will lead to high blood pressure in genetically predisposed persons. These facts have prompted many health organizations to advise against a high salt intake. Accordingly, we have reduced the amount of salt in recipes as much as possible, often by one-half. Instead, we are using herbs and spices abundantly.

If you want to reduce sodium further, use one of the many salt substitutes now on the market. These contain either no sodium or half the amount of sodium of table salt. Certainly do not add salt to already salted dishes at home or in restaurants.

Diverse low sodium or salt-reduced commercial products are now available in the supermarkets; notably tomato products, tomato sauces, creamed soups, and soy sauces. Use those in cooking; even though you may have to add some salt or salt substitute to the finished dish for taste, you will end up with food much lower in sodium than if you had used the regular commercial products.

Sugars

Neither white sugar nor any of the natural sweeteners have been linked with the development of cancer in human beings. Our concern here is that sugars are mostly a source of calories and may contribute to unwanted extra weight, a risk factor for cancer. We have simply cut down the amount of sugars in recipes by about one quarter or sometimes in half, or eliminated it when the small amount suggested did not affect the recipe one way or another. We have applied the same rule to all sources of sugars: white, brown, honey, or molasses.

In the introductory text we have sometimes suggested replacing butter or margarine with jams, jellies, or syrup. This is not a contradiction. In a cancer reducing diet, fats are worse than sugars and the above sugars are only suggested as improvements over fats in the very specific cases noted.

Fats

We have decreased the amounts of all sources of fat, including nuts, cheese, olives, and avocado, so that each recipe contains no more than about 2 teaspoons (10 grams) of fat per serving. We also have recommended that chicken be skinned before cooking to remove the layer of fat under the skin. We have used imitation mayonnaise instead of regular mayonnaise.

Fiber

The fiber content of recipes has been increased through the use of whole wheat flour and brown rice as well as liberal use of legumes, a variety of grains, vegetables, and fruit.

We are confident that these suggestions are in accord with the recommendations of many in the health field. We hope they help you follow a prudent diet while enjoying good food.

APPETIZERS & CONDIMENTS

Appetizers should tease and open the appetite, as their name suggests. Keep them as low in fat as possible. Avoid appetizers which include meat, poultry, or even fish. Save poultry, fish, and shellfish for the course of the dinner—unless the meal proper will be meatless.

Platters of raw vegetables are a good substitute for crackers to serve with dips. Use pureed beans, plain low fat yogurt, and low fat cottage cheese as bases for dips. Vegetables marinated in vinegar or lemon juice and herbs or spices will jolt the appetite.

SPICED CHEESE

1 cup low fat cottage cheese
3 tablespoons plain, low fat
   yogurt
1 tablespoon scallions or chives,
   chopped

1 tablespoon parsley
¼ teaspoon dried thyme
Freshly ground black pepper

Place all ingredients in blender or food processor. Blend thoroughly.
Serve on low fat crackers or use as dip for fresh vegetables. A salad
dressing can be made by thinning cheese mixture with yogurt. Yields
about 1½ cups.

⚜

FANCY & FRESH COCKTAIL POTATOES

Small red new potatoes
Plain low fat yogurt or low fat
   cottage cheese

Garnishes:
Chives
Olives
Chopped parsley
Pimientos
Green onions

Use potatoes of a similar size. Boil in water or steam until potatoes can be
pricked with a fork but are still firm. Drain. Cool. Cut each potato in half
and scoop out the middle with a melon ball tool. If using cottage cheese,
puree in food processor or blender. Fill center of each potato half with a
small dollop of yogurt or low fat cottage cheese and top with any
number of garnishes. Allow 3 potato halves per person.

ANTIPASTO

½ pound carrots
1 zucchini
1 small head cauliflower
1 small bunch broccoli
1 green pepper
1 can (6 oz.) black olives, pitted
 and drained
1 jar (6 oz.) artichoke hearts,
 drained and quartered
1 pound cherry tomatoes
½ pound fresh mushrooms, sliced
 lengthwise

½ jar (13 oz.) medium-hot chili
 peppers, drained

Chili Sauce Dressing:
½ cup chili sauce (tomato based)
1 tablespoon oil
¼ cup lemon juice
¼ cup wine vinegar
2-3 cloves garlic, minced
½ teaspoon dry mustard
1 teaspoon dried oregano
1 teaspoon dried basil

Chop or slice carrots, zucchini, cauliflower, broccoli, and green pepper into attractive, bite-size pieces. Boil vegetables briefly until crisp-tender (5 minutes for carrots, 2 minutes for other). Drain. In a saucepan combine chili sauce, oil, lemon juice, vinegar, garlic, mustard, oregano, and basil. Bring to boiling point. While hot, pour over boiled and drained vegetables in large bowl. Toss gently, cool to room temperature, drain well and add remaining vegetables. (Drained dressing can be used elsewhere for a salad dressing.) Toss thoroughly and gently. Chill. Can be made several days ahead and kept chilled. Makes 32 one-half cup servings.

VEGETABLE DIP

2 cups small-curd low fat cottage
   cheese
2 tablespoons dill weed
1 tablespoon Beau Monde
   seasoning

1 tablespoon green onion, finely
   chopped
½ tablespoon parsley, finely
   chopped
½ tablespoon lemon juice

Puree cottage cheese in food processor or blender for 2-3 minutes until creamy. Add remaining ingredients and process until mixed. Place in bowl and refrigerate. Serve with bite-size vegetables. Yields 2 cups.

※

HUMMUS

2 cups garbanzo beans, home
   cooked or canned
¼ cup sesame tahini, home
   prepared or purchased

3-4 tablespoons tamari (soy sauce)

Prepare your own garbanzo beans by covering 2 cups dry beans with water and soaking overnight. Then cook at simmer until soft, which usually takes all day. Grind garbanzo beans in blender or food processor. Prepare sesame tahini by combining ⅓ cup dry sesame seeds, ¼ cup vegetable oil, and ¼ cup lemon juice. Combine ¼ cup tahini and the tamari with garbanzo beans in blender. Store remaining tahini in refrigerator for future use. Will store at least 2 weeks. Hummus may be used as a dip with low fat crackers or as a sandwich spread. Yields 2½ cups.

DILLY TUNA DIP

1 cup low fat cottage cheese
1 can water-packed tuna, drained
½ teaspoon crushed dill weed

2 green onions, sliced
Lemon juice to taste
Paprika

In processor puree cottage cheese until creamy. Add tuna, dill, and lemon juice and process. Stir in green onion. Place in serving bowl and refrigerate at least 1 hour. Sprinkle with paprika before serving with low fat crackers. Yields 1½ cups.

⚜

SPINACH-WRAPPED CHICKEN WITH DIP

2 whole chicken breasts, boned
and skinned
1 small can chicken broth
1 tablespoon soy sauce
3 tablespoons water
1 tablespoon Worcestershire
sauce
1 large bunch fresh spinach

Sweet and Sour Sauce:
½ cup cider vinegar
½ cup sugar
1 cup water
3 thin slices ginger, or to taste
1 tablespoon cornstarch,
dissolved in 1 teaspoon soy
sauce

Poach whole chicken breasts in the mixed liquids for about 15 minutes. Cool in broth; cut into bite-size chunks and set aside. Wash spinach thoroughly and place in colander. Pour boiling water over spinach to wilt it and set aside to cool. To assemble, roll each chicken chunk in a spinach leaf, tucking loose ends under to make a neat package. Secure leaf with toothpick and chill. Bring to room temperature to serve.

To make sauce, dissolve vinegar and sugar in water; add ginger. Boil for 2 minutes. Add cornstarch/soy sauce binder and cook until thickened. Serve with fruit or vegetable garnish. Yields 2 cups sauce and about 40 pieces of chicken.

LOW CALORIE SPINACH DIP

1 cup plain low fat yogurt
1 package frozen chopped
    spinach, thawed and drained
½ cup parsley, chopped
½ cup green onion, chopped
½ teaspoon dill weed (or more)

½ teaspoon seasoned salt
½ cup low fat cottage cheese,
    pureed to consistency of sour
    cream
3 tablespoons imitation
    mayonnaise

Combine ingredients. Mix well and refrigerate for at least 5 or 6 hours, or overnight so that flavors have time to blend. Yields about 3½ cups.

⚜

YOGURT/HONEY/SESAME DIP

1 cup plain low fat yogurt
2 tablespoons honey
2 tablespoons lightly toasted
    sesame seeds

⅛ teaspoon powdered ginger
    (optional)

Mix ingredients in a small bowl. Use as a dip for fruit or as a dressing for fruit salad. Yields about 1¼ cups.

EGGPLANT DIP

1 large eggplant, unpeeled and
   sliced in half lengthwise
1 cup parsley, minced
1 large garlic clove, minced
½ small onion, minced

½ teaspoon dried basil
½ teaspoon dried oregano
½ teaspoon dried dill weed
3 teaspoons lemon juice
Pepper to taste

Bake eggplant on baking sheet for 50-60 minutes at 350°, or until soft. Cool and peel. Puree eggplant in processor. Add remaining ingredients and process for 5 seconds, adjusting for taste. Place dip in bowl and refrigerate. Serve with bite-size raw vegetables or low fat crackers. Yields about 2 cups.

❧

COLD ASPARAGUS WITH WALNUTS

1½ pounds fresh asparagus tips
1 tablespoon chopped walnuts
   (medium fine)
1 tablespoon sesame oil

¼ cup cider vinegar
¼ cup soy sauce
¼ cup sugar
White pepper

Cook asparagus in boiling water for 6-7 minutes or steam until tender. Drain and arrange in serving dish. Combine remaining ingredients and pour over asparagus. Lift asparagus to coat with dressing, sprinkle with pepper, and chill prior to serving. Serves 4.

PEACH CHUTNEY

4 quarts fresh ripe peaches, pitted
   and coarsely chopped
2 pounds dark brown sugar
2 cups cider vinegar
1 cup chopped onions
3 cups (1 pound) dark raisins
4 tart apples, peeled, cored, and
   coarsely chopped

2 tablespoons mustard seeds
¼ cup minced fresh ginger
1½ tablespoons salt
2 tablespoons paprika
1 tablespoon cumin
Juice of 2 limes
Grated rind of 1 lime

Place peaches in large heavy pot. Cover with sugar and vinegar. Add remaining ingredients and simmer, uncovered, stirring occasionally, for 2-3 hours or until thick. Pour into sterilized jars. Store in cool dark place. Makes 6-8 pints.

⚜

MOCK SOUR CREAM

2 tablespoons skim milk
1 tablespoon lemon juice

1 cup low fat cottage cheese

Place all ingredients in a blender and mix on medium-high speed until smooth and creamy. Use as a sour cream substitute. This sauce may be added to hot dishes at the last moment. Or serve it cold, with the addition of flavoring or herbs, as a dressing for salad or a sauce for mousse. Yields 1¼ cups.

PICKLED GREEN BEANS

2 pounds green beans
3 cups water
1 cup white vinegar
2 tablespoons pickling salt

2 tablespoons dried dill weed
¼ teaspoon cayenne pepper
1 tablespoon mustard seed
4 cloves garlic, minced

Cut green beans to fit quart jars, if necessary. Boil 3 cups water, vinegar, salt, dill, pepper, mustard seed, and garlic to make brine. Cover beans with brine to within ½ inch of top of sterilized jars. Process 10 minutes in hot water bath. Yields 2 quarts.

🌿

PEAR RELISH

1 cup sugar
1 cup white vinegar
2 teaspoons salt
¼-½ teaspoon cayenne pepper
6 fresh pears, cored and finely
   chopped

3 green peppers, diced
1 sweet red pepper, diced
2 large onions, finely diced

Combine sugar, vinegar, salt, and cayenne pepper in large saucepan; bring to boil. Add pears, peppers, and onions; return to boil. Reduce heat and simmer 25 to 30 minutes or until mixture thickens; stir occasionally. Ladle into clean hot canning jars to within ⅛ inch of tops. Seal according to jar manufacturer's directions. Place jars on rack in canner. Process 10 minutes in boiling water bath, water 2 inches above jar tops. Remove jars from canner. Place on thick cloth on wire racks; cool away from drafts. After 12 hours, test lids for proper seal. Makes about 5 (½ pint) jars.

APPLE BUTTER

4 pounds apples (Jonathan or
winesap are best for flavor)
2 cups water or cider
¼ cup sugar (per cup of pulp, see
below)

1 teaspoon cinnamon
½ teaspoon cloves
¼ teaspoon allspice
Grated rind of 1 lemon
2 tablespoons lemon juice

Wash, remove stems, and quarter apples. Cook slowly in water or cider
about 1 hour, or until soft. Put mixture through a fine strainer. Add ¼
cup sugar per cup of pulp. Add spices and lemon juice. Cook over low
heat, stirring constantly, until sugar is dissolved. Continue to cook and
stir frequently until apple butter coats spoon. Pour into hot sterilized all-
purpose canning jars with a two-piece metal screw top lid. (No need to
add paraffin.) Pour to the rim. Screw lid tightly. Cool. Store in cool, dry
place. Makes about 5 pints.

Variations:
Peach or apricot butters can be made in the same manner as below—
with ⅓ cup sugar per cup of pulp. Plum butter will need ½ to ¾ cup
sugar per cup of pulp. Delete spices.

SOUPS

Whether elegant or simple, soups can satisfy the appetite with few calories. Soup can be served as a snack; for lunch or as a part of the dinner meal or as the main dinner course. Hot or cold, with exotic combinations of food or with any leftover vegetables, soups can make excellent contributions to a cancer prevention style of eating.

Homemade stock and broth are excellent bases for soup. A recipe for chicken broth has been included in the soup recipes. Any extra can be stored in the freezer for later use. Use reduced-sodium canned soups or broths if you use commercial products as a base.

If you make soups at home from fresh vegetables, you can make a large quantity and refrigerate or freeze it.

BEAN & BASIL SOUP

1 cup potato, diced
2 cups carrot, diced
2 cups onion, diced
3 quarts water
1 teaspoon salt (optional)
1 cup uncooked macaroni
2 cups fresh green beans or 2
    packages (10 oz. each) frozen

1 can (16 oz.) cooked white beans,
    drained
3 cloves garlic, mashed
2 tablespoons fresh basil or 2
    teaspoons dried
4 tablespoons tomato paste
⅓ cup grated Parmesan cheese
1 tablespoon oil

Cook potatoes, carrots and onions in 3 quarts salted water until almost tender. Add green beans and macaroni; cook until tender.

In separate bowl, combine garlic, basil, tomato paste, and cheese; very slowly beat in the oil. Slowly add about 2 cups of the hot soup, beating vigorously. Pour the mixture back into the soup and mix well. Add the cooked white beans; heat through and serve hot. Serves 6.

⚜

BARLEY SOUP

2 cups pearl barley
4 cubes, or 1 tablespoon, chicken
    bouillon
1 carrot, thinly sliced

1 stalk celery, thinly sliced
½ medium onion, diced
1 bay leaf
6 cups water

Place barley in large cooking pot and add water to cover. Let stand overnight. The next day, combine remaining ingredients in the pot with barley and water. Add 6 cups water. Simmer for 2 hours. Serves 8.

COLD CUCUMBER SOUP

4 cups plain low fat yogurt
¼ cup walnuts, chopped
2 cups cucumbers, peeled and
   diced

White pepper to taste
1 tablespoon lemon juice
2 cloves garlic, crushed

Beat yogurt until smooth. Combine the remaining ingredients, add to yogurt, mixing well. Chill. Garnish with fresh mint, parsley, or coriander. Serves 4-6.

⚓

SHERRIED MUSHROOM SOUP

4 teaspoons margarine
½ cup scallions, finely chopped
2 cups mushrooms, thinly sliced
4 teaspoons all-purpose flour
⅛ teaspoon white pepper

1¼ quarts water
4 packets instant chicken broth
   and seasoning mix
4 teaspoons dry sherry

In 2-quart saucepan heat margarine over medium heat until bubbly and hot; add scallions and sauté, stirring occasionally, for 3 minutes. Add mushrooms and sauté until softened, about 3 minutes. Add flour and pepper and cook, stirring constantly for 1 minute. Continue to stir while adding water and broth mix and bring to a boil. Reduce heat to low, cover, and let simmer for 5 minutes. Stir in sherry and let simmer 2 minutes longer. Serves 8.

FASSOLADA (GREEK BEAN SOUP)

1 pound navy beans
2 teaspoons baking soda
2 tablespoons olive oil
1 large onion, chopped
2 cloves garlic, minced
2 large carrots, sliced

½ cup parsley, chopped
2 stalks celery and the leaves,
    chopped
1 can (16 oz.) tomatoes, chopped
Water
Pepper to taste

Soak beans in cold water overnight with baking soda. Pour out water and rinse. Add fresh water to cover well and bring to a boil. Boil vigorously for 20 minutes and discard water. Heat olive oil in pot. Sauté vegetables, except tomatoes, until transparent and lightly colored. Do not brown. Add beans and tomatoes, then add water. Pepper to taste. Cook slowly until beans are tender, about 1 hour. Add more water as necessary to keep beans covered. Serves 6.

🌱

SPRINGTIME VEGETABLE SOUP

1 tablespoon margarine or oil
3 bunches scallions, chopped
2 cups carrots, thinly sliced
2 cups fresh or frozen peas

4 stalks asparagus, cut into ½-inch
    pieces
⅓ cup celery leaves, chopped
6 cups chicken stock or water

Sauté scallions in oil or margarine. Add all vegetables to stock or water. Simmer for 15 to 20 minutes. Serves 6.

FRIENDSHIP BEAN SOUP

2½ cups dry bean mixture (may use a combination of dried beans, lentils, split peas)
1 tablespoon salt
Juice of 1 lemon

1 small can green chiles
2 medium onions, chopped
1 large can tomatoes
3 cloves garlic, minced

Place bean mixture in large kettle, cover with water and salt, and soak overnight. Drain and rinse. Add 2 quarts of water and simmer 3-4 hours. Add remaining ingredients and simmer 45 minutes. Serves 6-8.

☙

MINESTRONE DI OREGON SOUP

2 tablespoons olive oil
1 cup onion, thinly sliced
1 cup carrots, diced
1 cup celery, diced
2 cups potatoes, peeled and diced
3 cups cabbage, shredded
⅔ cup canned Italian tomatoes

3 cups seasonal vegetables, such as zucchini, green beans, peas, broccoli, all chopped
3 cups beef broth
3 cups water
1½ cups canned or cooked white beans

Sauté onion in oil. Add carrots and cook a few minutes. Repeat this procedure with the celery, potatoes, and vegetables, cooking each a few minutes and stirring. Add shredded cabbage. Add the tomatoes, broth, and water. Cover and cook over low heat for 3 hours until soup is thick. Add beans and simmer for 15 minutes. Serves 6-8.

SPLIT PEA VEGETABLE SOUP

1 cup dried split peas
2 cups water
2 tablespoons oil
½ onion, chopped
6-8 sprigs parsley, chopped
2 carrots, cut in rounds
2 stalks celery, chopped

2 tablespoons tomato sauce
2 bouillon cubes
6-7 cups water and bean juice
¼ head cabbage, chopped
¾ cup rice, uncooked
2 tablespoons Parmesan cheese to
garnish

Cook split peas in 2 cups water until soft. Sauté onions in oil until limp; add parsley and cook a few minutes. Add cooked split peas, water, and rest of ingredients except rice. Cook about 1 hour. Add rice and cook about 20 minutes, stirring frequently. If soup gets too thick, add more water or broth. Garnish with Parmesan cheese. Serves 6-8.

ॐ

ONION WINE SOUP

2 tablespoons margarine
5 large onions, chopped
3 cups chicken broth
2 cups water
½ cup celery leaves, chopped
1 large potato, sliced
1 cup dry white wine

1 tablespoon vinegar
1 teaspoon sugar
1 cup plain low fat yogurt or
nonfat milk
1 tablespoon parsley, minced
Dash of pepper

Melt margarine in a large saucepan. Add chopped onion and mix well. Add chicken broth, water, celery leaves, and potato. Bring to boiling. Cover and simmer for 30 minutes. Puree mixture in a blender. Return to saucepan and blend in wine, vinegar, and sugar. Bring to boiling and simmer for 5 minutes. Stir in yogurt or milk, parsley, and pepper to taste. Heat thoroughly but do not boil. Serves 6-8.

QUICK CHICKEN BROTH

Chicken bones and discarded
   carcass, cut up
2 or 3 cups water

1 bay leaf
1 sliced onion
Any favorite spices (optional)

Place discarded carcass and bones in 2 or 3 cups of water together with bay leaf, sliced onion, and any other spices. Boil for 15 minutes and strain. Broth can be stored in the refrigerator for 3-4 days or may be frozen.

❧

GAZPACHO

1 large onion, chopped
2 medium cucumbers, chopped
1 large can tomato juice
3 cloves garlic
2 cans chicken broth (refrigerate,
   then skim off fat before
   adding)
¼ cup red wine vinegar

1 teaspoon sugar
1 teaspoon salt

Garnishes:
Chopped green onion
Chopped cucumber
Chopped tomato
Chopped green pepper

Blend onion, cucumbers, tomato juice, and garlic in blender until smooth. Add chicken broth, vinegar, sugar, and salt and mix well. Chill and serve with any or all of the garnishes. Gazpacho without garnishes will keep for 2 weeks in refrigerator. Serves 8-10.

CHILI

1 pound pinto beans, sprouted
   3-4 days
4 cups tomatoes
1 large jalapeno pepper
1 medium onion

2 cloves garlic
Kelp to taste
Vegetable seasoning to taste
Oregano to taste
Chili powder to taste

Cook beans slowly over low heat. Put tomatoes, jalapeno, onion, and garlic through food grinder. Add kelp, vegetable seasoning, oregano, and chili powder to taste. Before serving add the hot beans to the raw vegetables with enough liquid to make the right consistency. Serves 4.

⚜

HEARTY TACO SOUP

½ pound extra lean ground beef
1 green pepper, diced
1 medium onion, diced
3 cups hot water
2 beef bouillon cubes
1 can (16 oz.) tomatoes, chopped,
   and liquid
1 can (15 oz.) small pinto beans
1 can (15 ¼ oz.) whole kernel
   corn

4 teaspoons chili powder
1 teaspoon cumin
¼ teaspoon garlic powder
⅛ to ¼ teaspoon cayenne pepper
6 crisp taco shells
¼ cup part-skim mozzarella
   cheese, grated

Brown meat in Dutch oven with green pepper and onion until beef is no longer pink; drain juices from pan. Dissolve bouillon cubes in hot water. Add to beef with tomatoes, beans, corn, chili powder, cumin, garlic powder, and cayenne pepper. Cover and simmer 30 minutes. Adjust seasonings to taste. Crumble 1 taco shell in each bowl; add soup and top with grated cheese. Serves 6.

SALADS & DRESSINGS

It is difficult to think of a food that cannot be eaten in a salad. Salads are an easy way to incorporate foods rich in vitamin A and C, such as vegetables and fruits, in your daily diet, whether in a meal or as a snack.

Peas or beans added to salads provide fiber and protein. Potato, rice, pasta, and bean salads, with or without animal foods, can easily be considered main dishes, replacing meat dishes. If you choose to use meat, poultry, or fish, remember that 1 or 2 ounces can go a long way.

If you use a salad dressing, be sure it is low in fat. Besides the dressing recipes, you will find ideas for dressings in the salad recipes.

LUNCH SALAD

½ cup raw carrots, grated
1 small shredded apple
½ teaspoon cinnamon

1 teaspoon imitation mayonnaise
1 teaspoon sugar

Toss all ingredients together. Makes 2 one-half-cup servings.

‎ 🌿

CHINESE CHICKEN SALAD

½ pound (3 breasts) chicken
⅓ cup soy sauce
⅓ cup sugar
¼ cup water
1 head iceberg lettuce
4 green onions
2 teaspoons almonds, chopped
2 teaspoons sesame seeds, toasted
2 ounces wonton wrappers
   (available at Oriental markets,
   as is mei-fun)

2 tablespoons oil
2 ounces (or more) mei-fun (rice
   stick)

Dressing:
2 tablespoons sugar
1 teaspoon salt
½ teaspoon pepper
1 tablespoon salad oil
½ teaspoon sesame oil
4 tablespoons white vinegar

Skin and bone chicken. Chop into small pieces and place in soy sauce/sugar/water mixture. Bake in 375° oven for 1 hour. Cool. Mix chicken in a large bowl along with the chopped green onions, almonds, toasted sesame seeds. Cut the wonton wrappers in strips and sauté in hot oil until brown. Remove and pat dry on paper towels. Drop mei-fun in hot oil (be ready to take it out quickly, as it cooks in just a few seconds). Add wonton, mei-fun, and torn lettuce to bowl. Top with the dressing. Serves 6.

CHICKEN SALAD A LA YOGURT

2 cups diced, cooked chicken
1 can (6 oz.) mushrooms, sliced
¼ cup tarragon vinegar
1 tablespoon salad oil
2 tablespoons minced onions
½ teaspoon salt

⅛ teaspoon pepper
¼ teaspoon thyme
⅛ teaspoon coriander (optional)
½ cup plain low fat yogurt
1 stalk celery, diced
Salad greens

Drain liquid from mushrooms. Combine vinegar, oil, onion, ¼ tsp. salt, and seasonings. Pour over mushrooms. Marinate several hours or overnight. Drain marinade from mushrooms. Mix yogurt with remaining ¼ teaspoon salt. Toss with chicken, celery, and mushrooms. Serve on salad greens. Serves 4.

❧

FRUITED CHICKEN SALAD

4 cups cooked chicken, diced
2 cups fresh pineapple, diced
1 can (12 oz.) mandarin oranges,
    drained
½ cup celery, chopped
½ cup green pepper, chopped

2 tablespoons onion, diced
1 cup imitation mayonnaise
    (optional)
1 tablespoon prepared mustard
    (optional)

Combine chicken, pineapple, oranges, celery, green pepper, and onion. If desired, mix mayonnaise and mustard and toss gently with chicken mixture. Cover and chill several hours or overnight. Serve in lettuce-lined bowls. Serves 8.

WILD RICE SALAD

½ cup wild rice
½ cup long-grain white rice
1 lemon slice
1 medium-sized carrot, peeled,
    trimmed, and diced
½ cup green peas (frozen may be
    used)
1 stalk celery, washed and thinly
    sliced
½ green pepper, cored, seeded,
    and diced

½ red pepper, cored, seeded, and
    diced
3 green onions, washed,
    trimmed, and thinly sliced

Vinaigrette Dressing
4 tablespoons cider vinegar
1 teaspoon Dijon mustard
2 tablespoons safflower oil
½ teaspoon dried thyme
Chopped parsley, to garnish

Soak the wild rice in hot water for 1 hour. Drain. Bring 1½ cups water to a
boil, add the wild rice, and cook over medium heat about 20 minutes.
Drain the rice using a colander and rinse quickly with hot water, shaking
occasionally. Bring 1 cup water to a boil, add the long-grain white rice
and the lemon, and cook over medium heat for 20 minutes. Drain the
rice using a colander and rinse quickly with hot water. Let the rice drain
thoroughly. Combine the wild rice and white rice together in a large
bowl. Set aside.

Prepare the vegetables, keeping them in separate bowls. Cook the
carrots in enough boiling water just to cover for 8-10 minutes or until just
tender. Drain and rinse with cold water. Blanch the peppers separately in
boiling water for 1 minute, drain, and refresh with cold water. Add all
the vegetables to the rice and mix together. In a small bowl mix vinegar
and mustard. Add the oil, drop by drop, whisking the entire time. Stir in
the thyme. At least an hour before serving, stir the vinaigrette into the
rice and vegetable mixture. Serve in a clear glass bowl. Garnish with
chopped parsley. Serves 6-8.

TUNA MACARONI SALAD

3 cups corkscrew macaroni,
   cooked (2 cups uncooked)
1 envelope (1¾ oz.) au gratin
   sauce
¾ cup water
½ cup low fat milk
¼ cup imitation mayonnaise
¼ teaspoon pepper

1 small zucchini, sliced
1 can (12½-13 oz.) water-packed
   tuna, drained
1 cup frozen peas
2 large stalks celery, sliced
2 green onions, minced
1 medium tomato, sliced

Mix all ingredients together and serve on lettuce. Serves 8-10.

🌿

MIMI'S TUNA SALAD

2 cups uncooked fettuccine
   noodles (curly spinach noodles
   or other vegetable non-egg
   noodles are colorful to use)
1 can water-packed tuna, drained
1 stalk celery, diced
1 can water chestnuts, diced

1 can jalapeno peppers, minced
4 green onions, diced
½ cup low fat plain yogurt
¼ cup imitation mayonnaise
1 tablespoon soy sauce
½ teaspoon garlic powder
½ teaspoon parsley flakes

Cook and drain noodles. Combine tuna, noodles, celery, water chestnuts, peppers, and onions. Combine yogurt and mayonnaise with soy sauce, garlic powder, and parsley to make a sauce. Combine all ingredients and toss lightly. Serve chilled. Serves 4.

SUNSHINE SPINACH SALAD

4 cups lettuce or other salad
   greens, torn
4 cups fresh spinach, torn
1 can (11 oz.) mandarin orange
   sections, drained, or 1 fresh
   orange, sliced
1 can (8 oz.) water chestnuts,
   drained and sliced

1 cup fresh mushrooms, sliced
1 small red onion, sliced and
   separated into rings
1 cup commercial low calorie
   Italian dressing

In large bowl, combine all ingredients except dressing. Chill until serving
time. Toss with dressing. Serves 6-8.

♣

SPINACH SALAD
WITH CURRY YOGURT DRESSING

2 bunches fresh spinach, washed
   and chilled
1 cup plain low fat yogurt
½ teaspoon salt

¼ teaspoon celery seeds
½ teaspoon garlic powder
⅛ teaspoon pepper
½ teaspoon curry powder

Break spinach into bite-size pieces in salad bowl. Combine remaining
ingredients. Pour over spinach, toss lightly to mix. Serves 6.

SPINACH ORANGE SALAD

2 tablespoons white wine vinegar
   or rice vinegar
1 tablespoon dry white wine
2 tablespoons safflower oil
1 teaspoon soy sauce
½ teaspoon sugar
½ teaspoon dry mustard
½ teaspoon curry powder

¼ teaspoon fresh ground pepper
1 large bunch spinach, washed
   and trimmed
2 oranges, peeled and cut into
   segments
Optional: diced green apple,
   raisins, green onions

Combine vinegar, wine, oil, soy sauce, sugar, dry mustard, curry powder, and pepper. Mix well with wire whisk. Pour dressing over spinach and toss well. Add orange segments and toss again. Any of the optional ingredients may be added to the salad before serving. Serves 4.

⚘

MOLDED SALAD

1 envelope unflavored gelatin
¼ cup cold water
¾ cup crushed water-packed
   pineapple
1 cup fresh frozen cranberries,
   coarsely ground while frozen

¼ cup sugar
½ cup orange juice
½ cup pineapple juice

Soften gelatin in water. Drain pineapple and measure ½ cup juice to be used in recipe. Combine cranberries, pineapple, and sugar and heat to almost boiling. Stir into gelatin and add juices. Pour into mold and chill to set. Serves 6.

MOLDED FRUIT SUMMER SALAD

2 packages (3 oz. each) orange
    gelatin
2 cups boiling water
1 pint orange sherbet

1½ cups fresh pineapple, diced
1 can (11 oz.) mandarin oranges,
    drained

Dissolve gelatin in water. Add sherbet, blend well. Chill until slightly thickened. Fold in pineapple and oranges. Turn into a 2-quart mold. Chill until firm. Unmold and garnish as desired. Serves 8-10.

         ⚓

CHILI BEAN SALAD

1 can (15 oz.) red kidney beans
1 can (15 oz.) pinto beans
1 can (15 oz.) garbanzo beans
1 can (15 oz.) whole kernel corn
½ cup green onions, chopped
¼ cup parsley, chopped
1 cup celery, sliced
1 can (4 oz.) green chiles, diced

Dressing:
2 tablespoons oil
¼ cup vinegar
1-2 cloves garlic, minced
1 teaspoon chili powder
1 teaspoon leaf oregano
¼ teaspoon ground cumin
⅛-½ teaspoon pepper or taco
    sauce (to taste)

Drain and rinse beans and corn. Combine all ingredients. Pour dressing over salad, mix well, and chill 6 hours or overnight (stirring several times). Serves 10.

PASTA BROCCOLI SALAD

2 cups cooked, drained pasta, any
  shape
1 large bunch broccoli, peeled,
  stems sliced, tops divided into
  florets
1 large red pepper, seeded and
  sliced
¼ cup French or Italian olives,
  seeded and halved

Dressing:
1 clove garlic, pressed
1 teaspoon dry mustard
2 tablespoons lemon juice
2 tablespoons parsley, minced
1 tablespoon fresh basil, chopped,
  or ½ teaspoon dry basil
⅓ cup white wine vinegar
2 tablespoons olive oil

In a large bowl combine pasta, broccoli, pepper, and olives. Whisk all
dressing ingredients together and toss with pasta and vegetable mixture.
Serve slightly chilled. Serves 4-6.

❧

TABOOLEY

1 cup cracked bulgur wheat
2 cups water
3 lemons, juice only
¼ cup olive oil
1 bunch green onions, chopped,
  including tops

2 large bunches parsley, chopped
½ cup fresh mint leaves, chopped
4 tomatoes, chopped

Soak wheat for at least 30 minutes. Drain off excess water and squeeze
dry. Blend lemon juice and oil together into wheat. Refrigerate several
hours or overnight. Add chopped vegetables to wheat mixture and chill
several hours before serving. This is a very attractive presentation when
served in a glass bowl. Serves 8-10.

CRANBERRY SALAD

2 cans (16 oz. each) cranberry
  sauce
2 envelopes plain gelatin
½ cup cold water

2 small cans mandarin oranges,
  drained
2 ounces nuts, chopped

Crush cranberry sauce with fork. Heat in top of a double boiler until dissolved. Soften gelatin in cold water. Add to hot cranberry sauce and stir until dissolved. Add oranges and nuts. Pour into mold and chill until firm. Serves 10-12.

⚜

CRANBERRY RELISH SALAD

2 cups raw cranberries
1 large apple, cored
1 large orange and rind

¾ cup sugar
2 cups fresh pineapple, diced
¼ cup nuts, chopped

Grind in food processor or hand food grinder first 3 ingredients with juice, apple peel, and orange rind. Add the sugar, pineapple, and nuts. Mix well and chill in refrigerator. Serve as a raw salad or a relish. Good with roast turkey. Serves 8.

BULGUR CABBAGE SALAD

½ cup bulgur wheat
1 cup water
½ teaspoon salt
½ cup imitation mayonnaise
3 tablespoons cider vinegar
2 tablespoons sugar
¼ teaspoon liquid hot pepper
seasoning (optional)

¼ teaspoon dill weed (optional)
¼ teaspoon Dijon mustard
(optional)
½ cup green onion, thinly sliced
1½ cup cabbage, finely shredded
½ cup celery, thinly sliced
½ cup carrot, shredded

In a saucepan, combine bulgur, water, and salt; bring to a boil, stir, cover, and simmer for 15 minutes. Stir together mayonnaise, vinegar, sugar, green onion, and optional seasonings, if desired. Blend dressing into the hot cooked bulgur, cover and chill well. About 1 hour before serving, combine the bulgur with the cabbage, celery, and carrot; blend well. Spoon mixture into a salad bowl, cover and chill until serving time. Serves 4-6.

⚘

FRESH FRUIT SALAD

1 pint fresh strawberries,
stemmed and sliced
2 bananas, peeled and sliced
1 each sweet red and tart green
apple, cored and chopped
(leave peels on)

1 can pineapple chunks in own
juice, drained. Save juice.
2 fresh oranges, peeled and
segmented
½ cup mini-marshmallows
(optional)

Prepare fruit as directed and toss gently with pineapple juice to coat fruit thoroughly. Chill. Add marshmallows prior to serving. Serves 4-6.

PEAR SHRIMP SALAD

3 fresh winter pears
Salad greens
1 pound cooked tiny shrimp
1 cup chopped celery
⅓ cup chopped green pepper

¼ cup chopped green onion
¼ cup imitation mayonnaise
½ teaspoon curry powder
¼ teaspoon salt

Core pears and cut into wedges. Arrange on lettuce-lined salad plates. Combine shrimp, celery, green peppers, and green onion. Blend mayonnaise, curry powder, and salt. Toss with shrimp mixture. Add to salad plates with pears. Serves 6.

⚜

CHERYL'S RAINBOW SALAD

8 cups red and green cabbage,
    shredded
1 can (11 oz.) mandarin oranges,
    drained
1 red apple, diced
1 green apple, diced

1 green pepper, diced
¼ cup walnut bits
½ teaspoon celery seed
1 cup plain low fat yogurt
½ cup V-8 juice

In a large clear glass salad bowl, combine all fruits, vegetables, walnuts, and celery seed. Mix well and then add yogurt and juice. Refrigerate 2 hours, then toss again before serving chilled. Serves 4-6.

LOW CALORIE SAVORY SALAD DRESSING

3 cups water, boiling
2½ boxes pectin
½ cup red wine vinegar
¼ cup tarragon vinegar
¾ cup tomato juice
½ teaspoon dry mustard

⅛ teaspoon thyme
½ teaspoon white pepper
½ teaspoon paprika
2 tablespoons grated onion
1½ teaspoons sugar

Add pectin to boiling water and stir to mix. Cook 1 minute. Remove from heat and add remaining ingredients. Blend thoroughly. Chill. Store covered in refrigerator. Beat well or shake vigorously before serving. Yields 1 quart.

❧

SOY SALAD DRESSING

1 teaspoon oil
1 garlic clove, minced
1 slice ginger, minced
1 scallion, sliced

¼ cup low sodium soy sauce
2 tablespoons rice vinegar
1 tablespoon sugar
¼ teaspoon sesame oil

Combine all ingredients. This recipe is good with chicken salad. Yields about ½ cup.

BREADS & CEREALS

In making bread that is meant to reduce the risk of cancer, whole wheat flour is used, alone or mixed in equal parts with white flour. Also, fat is reduced—no more than 2 teaspoons per serving, amounts of whole eggs are reduced, and skim milk is recommended. Greater use is made of vegetables and fruits in the making of the breads. These flavorful breads do not need any spread or topping.

We often think of cereals as breakfast foods, when really they are grains, such as oats, rice, and corn, suitable for eating anytime. And bran is a cereal made from the husks removed when grain is refined. In this section you will find recipes that make use of cereals for breakfast food. Other recipe sections also include grains.

100% WHOLE WHEAT BREAD

1 package dry yeast
¼ cup warm water
2 cups low fat milk, scalded
¼ cup sugar

¼ cup molasses
3 tablespoons oil
3 teaspoons salt
5 cups whole wheat flour

Soften yeast in warm water. Add sugar, molasses, oil, and salt to scalded milk and stir to blend. Pour into large mixing bowl and cool to luke-warm. Stir in softened yeast. Add flour, beating until well mixed. Turn dough onto floured surface and knead 8-10 minutes, until smooth and elastic. Place in oiled bowl, turning to oil surface. Cover and let rise in warm place until double. Punch down, divide dough into 2 equal parts, and shape into loaves. Place in 2 greased, large bread pans and let rise until double. Bake at 400° for 20-25 minutes.

⚜

NO-KNEAD WHEAT BREAD

7 cups stone-ground whole
    wheat flour
6 tablespoons wheat germ
1 teaspoon salt

½ cup honey
3½ cups very warm water
2 tablespoons yeast
1 cup lukewarm water

Mix flour, wheat germ, and salt. Dissolve honey in very warm water; stir into flour (a little at a time). Dissolve yeast in lukewarm water; stir into flour mixture. Spoon into 2 well-greased 8½ x 4½ bread pans. Let rise for 30 minutes. Bake at 350° for 45 minutes. Makes 2 loaves.

WHOLE WHEAT FRENCH BREAD

1 tablespoon active dry yeast
1 tablespoon sugar
1 teaspoon salt (or less)
2½ cups lukewarm water

3 cups white flour
2-3 cups whole wheat flour
1 egg white mixed with 1
    tablespoon cold water

Combine yeast, sugar, salt, and water in a large bowl. Gradually add the flours and mix well (hands work best). At first the dough will be very sticky: add enough flour to transfer it to a lightly floured board. Knead until no longer sticky (about 10 minutes), adding more flour as necessary. Place in lightly oiled bowl. Cover with a damp cloth and let rise in warm place until doubled in volume. (1 ½-2 hours).

Punch dough down. Transfer to a floured board and cut into four equal parts. Roll and shape each part into a long loaf. Place loaves into lightly oiled special long loaf pans (baguette pans). Slash the top of each loaf diagonally in three or four places and brush with the egg white and water mixture. Preheat oven to 350°. Let dough rise another hour, or until doubled in volume. Bake until browned and hollow sounding when thumped (25 minutes). Halfway through baking, it may be necessary to cover the loaves with aluminum foil to prevent scorching the tops. Let cool on racks. Makes 4 loaves about 18 inches long.

If planning to freeze bread, bake only 15 minutes. Wrap in foil when cool. When ready to serve, remove from freezer, leave wrapped in foil. Place in 350° oven for 10 minutes. Remove foil and continue to bake for 5 minutes, until crisp.

WHOLE WHEAT RAISIN BREAD

3 cups whole wheat flour
¼ cup toasted wheat germ
2 teaspoons baking powder
1¼ teaspoons soda
1 teaspoon salt

1½ cups buttermilk
½ cup honey
¼ cup oil
½ cup raisins

Combine the dry ingredients in a large bowl. Separately combine the liquids and add all at once to the dry mixture with the raisins. Mix until just blended—do not overmix. Pour batter into 8½ x 4½ loaf pan that has been sprayed with cooking spray and bake at 325° for 1¼ hours.

🌿

CARROT BREAD

2 cups orange juice
2 teaspoons sugar
1 package yeast
¼ cup honey
¼ cup oil
2 teaspoons salt

4 cups whole wheat flour
2 cups carrots, grated
2 eggs, or 1 egg and 2 egg whites
1 cup rye flour
1 cup white flour

Warm the orange juice and stir in sugar and yeast. Combine oil, salt, and honey. Add 1 cup whole wheat flour, carrots, and eggs, and combine well. Gradually add the rye and white flour, then enough remaining wheat flour to make a stiff dough. Knead the dough and let rise until doubled in volume. Punch down, divide into 2 equal parts, and place in 8½ x 4½ loaf pans. Let bread rise again and bake at 350° for 45 minutes.

CARROT SANDWICH BREAD

1 cup raw carrots, finely grated
½ cup brown sugar
1 teaspoon baking soda
1 tablespoon oil
1 cup boiling water
1 egg or 2 egg whites

2½ teaspoons baking powder
½ teaspoon salt
1½ cups all-purpose flour, sifted
1 cup whole wheat flour
¼ cup walnuts, chopped

Combine carrots, sugar, baking soda, and oil in a large bowl. Pour on the boiling water and stir just to mix. Set aside to cool. Beat egg with a fork and add to the cooled carrot mixture. Sift in the baking powder, salt, and all-purpose flour. Stir in the whole wheat flour. Fold in walnuts. Pour into an oiled 8½ x 4½ loaf pan. Let stand 5 minutes.

Bake in moderate (350°) oven for 1 hour. Remove from pan and cool on wire rack. Bread slices better if allowed to stand, wrapped in foil or plastic wrap, in a cool place overnight. Makes 1 loaf.

⚜

OATMEAL BREAD

1⅛ cups oatmeal, uncooked
1 teaspoon salt
¼ cup molasses
4 tablespoons margarine, melted

2 cups boiling water
1 package yeast
⅓ cup warm water
5½ cups flour

Combine oatmeal, salt, molasses, and margarine in a large bowl. Stir in boiling water and let stand until cool. Dissolve yeast in ⅓ cup warm water and add to oat mixture. Add flour and knead thoroughly. Let rise until double in bulk. Knead down and form 2 loaves. Let rise again. Bake at 375° for 45 minutes. Makes 2 loaves.

SOURDOUGH STARTER

1 cake or 1 package yeast
½ cup lukewarm water
2 cups flour

1 tablespoon salt
1 tablespoon sugar
1½ cups cold water

Soften yeast in ½ cup lukewarm water. Measure flour, salt, and sugar into a large bowl or crock (one large enough to allow the starter to bubble to four times its volume). Stir in softened yeast and cold water. Cover with tea towel and let stand in warm place (80° to 90° is ideal), stirring it down daily. In 3 to 4 days it should have pleasantly sour odor. The starter is now ready. Use it at once or cover tightly and refrigerate.

⚜

BUTTERMILK CORN BREAD

2 cups corn meal
½ cup wheat germ
½ teaspoon salt
½ teaspoon baking soda
1 teaspoon baking powder

1 tablespoon brown sugar
1 large egg or 2 egg whites
1 tablespoon oil
2 cups buttermilk
1 cup carrots, grated

Stir dry ingredients into a large bowl, set aside. Mix liquids. Combine with dry ingredients until well mixed. Turn into 8 x 8 baking pan, well greased, or use larger pan if you wish thinner cornbread. Bake in 425° oven for 25-30 minutes.

HARRY'S BAGELS

2 cups warm water
1½ tablespoons salt
1½ tablespoons sugar
2 tablespoons oil
2 envelopes dry yeast

¼ cup water, warm
2 eggs, beaten, or 1 whole egg
  and 2 whites
7-8 cups flour
Large pan boiling water

Pour warm water over salt, sugar, and oil. Add yeast that has been dissolved in ¼ cup warm water. Mix in the eggs and 4 cups flour and beat together thoroughly (use electric mixer). Add enough flour to make a stiff dough (about 3 or 4 more cups). Knead well. Place in lightly oiled bowl, turning to oil surface. Cover with cloth and place in warm spot to rise until double in bulk. This should take about 1½ hours.

Turn dough out of bowl onto floured board. Cut off pieces of dough about the size of ⅓ cup (one piece at a time). Roll with hand to size of middle finger (4 inches or more). Then place around hand at knuckles and roll ends together. Place on floured board. When formed, cover and let rise again for 15-20 minutes. Then drop into boiling water (3 or 4 at a time) for about ½ to 1 minute. Turn over briefly. Remove from water with a slotted spoon, place on oiled cookie sheet, and bake at 425° until light brown, about 15-20 minutes. Cool on racks. Makes 28-30 bagels.

❧

BUTTERMILK QUICK BREAD

3½ cups whole wheat flour
½ cup bran flour
1 tablespoon baking powder
¼ teaspoon salt
¼ teaspoon baking soda

¼ to ½ cup raisins
½ cup nuts (optional)
1 teaspoon honey
2 cups buttermilk, room
  temperature

Mix all ingredients, form into a ball, make a cross on the top. Place on well-greased pie tin. Bake at 425° for 45-50 minutes. Makes 1 loaf.

PITA BREAD

2 cups warm water   1 teaspoon salt
1 package yeast   4½ cups unsifted flour

Pour water into large bowl; add yeast and stir until dissolved. Add salt and gradually stir in the flour, beating until a smooth dough forms. Scrape dough down from sides of bowl, cover lightly, and let rise in a warm place until doubled (about 1 hour). Stir down and divide into 12 parts, placing them on a very well-floured board. Cover lightly and let stand for 30 minutes. Place 2 of the dough mounds on a lightly greased and floured cookie sheet. With fingers, press lightly around the edge of the dough to flatten and shape into rounds about 5 inches in diameter and about ½ inch thick. Try not to squeeze out air bubbles; instead, force them to the center of the bread.

With oven shelf at lowest possible level, bake in a moderate oven (350°) for 20 minutes. (Buns should puff up but not be browned.) When all buns are baked, place under the broiler for about 1 minute to brown tops lightly. This bread freezes well. Makes 12 buns.

⚜

IRISH SODA BREAD

2½ cups whole wheat flour   1½ teaspoons soda
1½ cups white flour   ¼ cup bran
1 tablespoon sugar   ¼ cup wheat germ
1 teaspoon salt   2 cups buttermilk

Mix all ingredients thoroughly, turn onto a floured bread board, and knead until smooth . . . the less the better. Divide into 2 loaves and bake in oiled 8½ x 4½ loaf pans for 45 minutes in 350° oven. Makes 2 loaves.

WHOLE WHEAT SUNFLOWER MUFFINS

½ cup white flour
2½ teaspoons baking powder
½ teaspoon salt
1½ cups whole wheat flour
¼ cup sunflower seeds, unsalted
1 egg or 2 egg whites
¾ cup low fat milk

⅓ cup corn oil
⅓ cup honey
Optional: ½ teaspoon cinnamon,
    sifted with dry ingredients, 1
    tablespoon grated orange peel,
    added to liquids

Sift white flour, baking powder, and salt. Add whole wheat flour and seeds. Mix well. Beat together egg, oil, milk, and honey. Add liquids all at once to dry ingredients. Stir just until dry ingredients are moistened. Fill oiled muffin cups ⅔ full. Bake at 400° approximately 15-20 minutes. Makes 12-14 muffins.

⚓

NATURAL BRAN MUFFINS

2 cups 100% bran
2 cups boiling water
5 cups unbleached flour
5 teaspoons baking soda
1 quart buttermilk
4 cups 40% bran flakes

1 teaspoon salt
3 cups sugar
¼ cup shortening
1 egg or 2 egg whites
1 cup mixed dried fruit with
    raisins (optional)

Mix bran and water, let cool. Sift flour and soda into mixing bowl. Add sugar, shortening, and egg. Blend well, add buttermilk and bran flakes. Fill ⅔ full each cup of two well-greased muffin tins. Bake at 400° for 20-25 minutes. Yields 5-6 dozen.

BRAN MUFFINS

½ cup oil
3⅔ cups plain dry bran flakes
2¾ cups buttermilk
¼ cup skim milk powder
1 cup brown sugar

½ cup honey
1 egg and 3 egg whites
3½ cups flour
3½ teaspoons baking soda

Pour oil and bran into a bowl and mix well. Let oil soak into bran for 6 hours or overnight. Place buttermilk in another bowl. Dissolve milk powder in buttermilk with hand whip. Dissolve honey, brown sugar, and eggs and add to the milk mixture. Stir until smooth. Sift flour then add soda, mixing well to distribute soda evenly. Pour the liquid ingredients into the bran and oil mixture in a large bowl. Stir until of uniform consistency. Add flour-soda mixture. Stir until of uniform consistency. Place in cupcake tins with paper liners or spray-coated pans. Bake at 350° for 20-25 minutes. Makes 2 dozen large or 3 dozen medium muffins.

ᴥ

FRUITED BRAN MUFFINS

1 cup bran flakes
1 cup bananas, mashed
1 cup raisins
1 egg

¼ cup oil
1 cup flour
2½ teaspoons baking powder
¼ cup sugar

Mix bran flakes, bananas, raisins, egg, and oil. Add flour, baking powder, and sugar; stir to moisten all. Do not overmix. Pour into muffin tins. Bake 25 minutes at 400°. Makes 12 muffins.

THREE-BRAN MUFFINS

½ cup dates or raisins
½ cup boiling water
1¼ teaspoons baking soda
3 tablespoons margarine
½ cup sugar
1 egg or 2 egg whites
1 cup buttermilk or low fat
  yogurt
1¼ cups flour (can use whole
  wheat flour)
½ cup 40% bran flakes

1 cup all-bran
¼ cup miller's bran
¼ cup chopped walnuts or
  sunflower seeds
¼ teaspoon salt
½ teaspoon cinnamon
Optional: 2 apples, peeled and
  chopped; 8 ounces pineapple,
  crushed and drained; 1 banana,
  mashed; 2 carrots, peeled and
  grated

Mix dates, boiling water, and baking soda. Stir and set aside to cool. Cream margarine, sugar, and egg. Add buttermilk and flour alternately. Stir in date mixture. Add bran flakes, all-bran, miller's bran. Combine well. Add nuts, salt, cinnamon, and one of optional ingredients. Beat on slow speed. Can be stored in refrigerator up to one week if desired. Bake at 375° for 20-25 minutes. Makes 12 large muffins.

⚘

BEST CORN-OAT WAFFLES

3 cups oatmeal, uncooked
½ cup cornmeal (non-
  degerminated is best)
¼ cup pitted dates

2 tablespoons sunflower seeds
¼ teaspoon salt
1 teaspoon vanilla
4 cups water

Mix all ingredients together in blender until smooth. Bake in preheated waffle iron for 5-10 minutes. Do not lift top too soon. These waffles rise by steam and are crisp and tender. Use fresh fruit, applesauce, and blueberries or other fruit as toppings. Serves 4.

OATMEAL PANCAKES

1½ cups low fat milk
1 cup rolled oats
1 tablespoon oil
1 egg or 2 egg whites
2 tablespoons water

½ cup whole wheat flour
1 tablespoon brown sugar
1 teaspoon baking powder
¼ teaspoon salt
1 cup blueberries or other fruit

Combine milk and rolled oats and let set for 5 minutes. Add oil, egg, and water; stir to blend. Add dry ingredients and stir just until moistened. Add blueberries or other fruit. Cook as regular pancakes. Makes 10 to 12 4-inch pancakes.

⁂

DR. GALEN'S BREAKFAST CHOICE

1 cup puffed wheat
2 ounces plain low fat yogurt
½ cup fresh fruit (berries, banana,
    pear, etc.)

3 tablespoons miller's bran
¾ cup skim milk

Start with the puffed wheat and add the other ingredients in order. Serves 1.

LOW FAT GRANOLA

⅓ cup oil
½ cup honey
¼ cup water
1 teaspoon vanilla extract
4½ cups rolled wheat
1 cup oatmeal

2 cups dry cereals such as Bran
   Flakes, 40% Bran, Wheaties
¼ cup sunflower seeds, hulled
¼ cup walnuts, chopped
½ cup nonfat milk powder
1 cup raisins or other dried fruit

In saucepan, heat oil, honey, water, and vanilla until blended. In large bowl, combine cereals, nuts, and milk powder. Pour liquid ingredients over dry ones and mix well. Spread mixture on 2 jelly roll pans. Bake at 350° for 10 minutes, stirring occasionally. Remove from oven; add raisins. Let cool until crisp, store in airtight container. Makes about 10 cups.

ᴥ

MILLET CEREAL

4 cups water
1 cup whole grain millet

⅓ cup raisins
⅛ teaspoon salt (optional)

Bring water to a boil with salt, if used. Add fruit and millet. Simmer on low setting with lid slightly ajar until millet becomes fluffy and water is absorbed—about 20-30 minutes. Serves 4.

VEGETABLES

Nature provides a large variety of vegetables from which to choose. In a low fat diet, vegetable dishes are not considered just side dishes: they are often main dishes. However you prepare them, serve two vegetables at lunch and at dinner. They make excellent snacks as well.

Raw vegetables are best, but we have included interesting recipes here for those who prefer them cooked. The emphasis is on mustard family vegetables, such as broccoli, and deep yellow vegetables.

BROCCOLI WITH ORANGE SAUCE

1 teaspoon margarine
1 teaspoon olive oil
1 clove garlic
1/3 cup orange juice, unsweetened

1/4 cup dry white wine
2 teaspoons grated orange peel
1 pound broccoli, trimmed
1/4 cup chopped green onions

Combine margarine and olive oil, sauté garlic until lightly browned. Add orange juice, peel, and wine. Boil on high until reduced by half. Meanwhile, steam broccoli until crisp-tender. Add chopped green onion to orange juice mixture; pour over broccoli. Serve immediately. Serves 4.

&

GLAZED CARROTS

1 tablespoon margarine
1 small onion, finely chopped
1 pound carrots, scrubbed and
   sliced 1 inch thick
2 tablespoons honey
1/8 teaspoon grated nutmeg

Chicken Stock:
Bony chicken pieces
1/2 cup chopped celery
1 carrot, grated
Salt

To make stock, simmer bony chicken pieces with 1/2 cup chopped celery, 1 grated carrot, and 1/2 teaspoon salt in 1 quart water until tender. Bone chicken to use later. Strain the broth and allow to cool. Remove the fat. Broth may be frozen in ice cube trays and used as needed.

Melt margarine in medium saucepan over medium-low heat. Add and sauté onion until limp. Add carrots and stock. Cover and cook over medium heat until carrots are tender (about 15 minutes). Then add honey and nutmeg. Continue to cook, stirring occasionally, until the remaining liquid becomes syrupy. Serves 4.

YIA YIA'S MUMBALDI

4 eggplants, quartered lengthwise
1 tablespoon margarine
5 onions, cut in slivers lengthwise
1 entire head garlic, peeled and
    sliced

1 large or 2 small tomatoes,
    chopped
Double handful fresh parsley or
    ¼ cup dried parsley

Brown eggplant in as little vegetable oil as possible. Arrange eggplant in a large, fairly deep baking dish, packing it tightly. Sauté in 1 tablespoon margarine the onion and garlic until the onion is limp. Arrange over eggplant. Put chopped tomato and parsley over eggplant. Add 1 inch water to pan. Bake at about 375° uncovered until the water is mostly gone. May be served hot, warm, or at room temperature. Serves 12-14.

♣

MARINATED VEGETABLES

1 cup carrot rounds
1 cup celery, sliced
1 cup cauliflower, sliced
1 cup broccoli florets
1 medium onion, sliced
1 green bell pepper, sliced
1 zucchini, sliced

Italian Dressing:
¼ cup olive oil
¾ cup vinegar (wine vinegar
    preferred)
1 tablespoon dry Italian seasoning
    mix
¼ teaspoon sugar
½ teaspoon pepper
1 teaspoon garlic powder
1 teaspoon onion powder

Clean and prepare vegetables. Place in 2-quart refrigerator dish. Mix dressing and pour over raw vegetables. Cover and refrigerate for 12 hours. Drain vegetables before serving. Serves 8.

MEXICAN VEGETABLES

1 tablespoon oil
1 onion, chopped
1 clove garlic, minced
1 hot fresh chili pepper, chopped;
    or ¼ cup green pepper,
    chopped, and ¼ teaspoon
    cayenne; or 1-2 teaspoons chili
    powder
2 cups fresh chopped or canned
    drained tomatoes

¼ teaspoon salt
4 cups diced vegetables, including
    cooked dried beans, corn,
    green beans, squash or
    cauliflower
2 tablespoons grated Parmesan
    cheese

Heat oil and sauté garlic, onion, and pepper about 5 minutes. Add tomatoes and salt and bring to a boil. Add vegetables, cover, and cook gently for about 30 minutes, depending on the vegetables. Serve over corn bread or other whole grain bread. Sprinkle with a little cheese. Serves 4.

⚜

OVEN-FRIED POTATOES

1 large potato

Preheat the oven to 400°. Scrub the potato well and cut in half lengthwise then cut into wedges. Spray a cookie sheet with non-stick cooking spray. Bake the potato wedges 15 minutes, loosen from pan and turn them, then bake another 10-15 minutes. Serves 1.

SPICED CAULIFLOWER

1 tablespoon oil
2 tablespoons finely chopped
  onion
1 small clove garlic, crushed
¼ teaspoon ground ginger
¼ teaspoon turmeric

2 whole cloves
1 head cauliflower, medium size
Dash salt
2 tablespoons toasted sliced
  almonds, or raisins

Heat oil in skillet. Add onions, garlic, ginger, turmeric, and cloves. Stir
and simmer for 5 minutes. Break cauliflower into separate florets. Cut
lengthwise in bite-size pieces, add to spices. Cover and shake to coat each
piece. Add 2 tablespoons water and dash of salt. Steam over medium-low
heat, shaking pan frequently. If needed, add more water. Cauliflower
should be tender in about 10 minutes. Garnish with almonds or raisins.
Serves 4.

⚜

CREAMED BRUSSELS SPROUTS

1 tablespoon plus 1 teaspoon
  margarine
½ cup onion, finely chopped
3 tablespoons all-purpose flour
1 cup each skim milk and water

2 packets instant chicken broth
  and seasoning mix
¼ cup ground nutmeg
4 cups brussels sprouts, cooked

In 2-quart saucepan heat margarine over medium heat until bubbly and
hot; add onion and sauté until softened. Add flour and cook, stirring
constantly for 1 minute; continue to stir, add milk, water, and broth mix
and bring to a boil. Reduce heat to low, add nutmeg, and cook, stirring
constantly, until mixture is smooth and thickened. Add sprouts and
cook, stirring constantly until thoroughly combined and heated. Transfer to serving plate and pour any remaining sauce over brussels sprouts.
Serves 8.

TANGY BLACK BEANS

1 large onion, chopped
2 cloves garlic, chopped
1 tablespoon oil
1 cup dry black beans
3 cups stock or water (or
  substitute wine for up to half
  of stock)

1 bay leaf
¼ teaspoon pepper
1 orange, whole or halved
½ teaspoon salt
2 stalks celery, chopped
1 tomato, chopped

Sauté the onion and garlic in a little oil, then add them to the beans, with stock, the bay leaf, and pepper. Bring to a boil, simmer 2 minutes, and let sit, covered, for 1 hour. Add the whole or halved orange (whole is the traditional way), salt, celery, and tomato. Simmer covered, with lid ajar, for 2 to 3 hours or more, until the beans are tender. Remove a ladleful of beans, mash them, and return them to the pot to cook until the mashed beans thicken the mixture. Excellent with rice. Serves 6.

🌱

MARINATED BROCCOLI

3 bunches fresh broccoli
1½ cups cider vinegar
1 tablespoon sugar
1 tablespoon dill weed

1 teaspoon salt
1 teaspoon pepper
1 teaspoon garlic powder
2 tablespoons oil

Slice broccoli into long pieces. Pour ingredients over and refrigerate 24 hours. Baste, drain, and serve. Serves 4-6.

HAZELNUT BROCCOLI

2 packages (10 oz. each) frozen
    broccoli (or 1½ lb. fresh,
    chopped)
2 tablespoons margarine
3 tablespoons flour
1 tablespoon powdered chicken
    stock base

1½ cups low fat milk
¼ cup water
1 cup herb stuffing mix
¼ cup roasted hazelnuts, coarsely
    chopped

Cook broccoli until tender, drain thoroughly, put into a slightly oiled 1½ quart casserole. In a saucepan, melt 1 tablespoon margarine, blend in flour and chicken stock base to make a smooth paste. Gradually add milk and cook, stirring frequently until thick and smooth. Mix into broccoli. Heat water and remaining 1 tablespoon margarine until melted; pour over stuffing mix and hazelnuts and toss. Top broccoli with hazelnut mixture. Bake, uncovered, at 400° for 20 minutes. Serves 6.

ىك

RATATOUILLE PROVENCALE

2½ cups cubed eggplant (½ inch)
¼ cup thinly sliced onion
2 cloves garlic, minced
1 tablespoon olive oil
4 green peppers, sliced

2 cups quartered tomatoes
3 cups sliced zucchini (½ inch
    thick)
1 teaspoon oregano leaves
Pepper to taste

Sauté onions and garlic in olive oil. Add green peppers, tomatoes, and zucchini; sauté until heated. Add eggplant, oregano, and pepper. Cook very slowly in covered dish about 15 minutes longer. May be served hot or cold. Serves 8.

HERBED BRUSSELS SPROUTS

1 pound Brussels sprouts
1 small onion, sliced
1 tablespoon margarine
1 clove garlic, minced
¼ teaspoon thyme

¼ teaspoon oregano
⅛ teaspoon salt
⅛ teaspoon pepper
¼ cup chopped parsley

Steam Brussels sprouts and onions 15 minutes or until tender. In a skillet, melt margarine and sauté garlic until slightly browned. Add Brussels sprouts, onion, and herbs except parsley. Gently stir and cook until vegetables are heated through. Sprinkle parsley over sprouts before serving. Serves 4.

⚜

DILL CABBAGE

⅓ cup chicken broth
4 cups cabbage, coarsely shredded
½ cup carrots, coarsely shredded
¼ cup sliced green onions
½ teaspoon dill

¼ teaspoon pepper
1 tablespoon margarine
1 tablespoon filberts, chopped
½ teaspoon mustard

In large saucepan, mix cabbage, carrots, green onions, dill, and pepper in chicken broth. Cook, covered, over medium heat until tender, about 5 minutes. Melt margarine and mix in filberts and mustard. Pour over vegetables. Serves 6.

POULTRY

Chicken and turkey hold a very high position in many cuisines of the world. Their delicate flesh and lower fat content make them a good choice of animal protein food for an eating style low in fat.

Poultry can often be used in dishes calling for red meat. Ground turkey, for example, makes an excellent replacement for ground beef.

Most of the fat in poultry is carried in a layer under the skin. So it is best to cook and eat chicken without the skin. Chicken blends well with many spices, so use them to replace the crunchy taste of the chicken skin with spices.

TAGGART'S SPICY CHICKEN WITH CASHEWS

1 pound boneless chicken,
trimmed of skin and fat

Velveting Mixture:
1 teaspoon salt
1 tablespoon dry sherry
1 egg white
1 tablespoon cornstarch
1 tablespoon oil

Aromatics:
2 cloves minced garlic
2 quarter-size sliced ginger,
minced
6 dried red chiles or ¾ teaspoon
crushed chiles
1 scallion, cut in ½-inch pieces
1 sweet red bell pepper, cut in
½-inch pieces

Sauce:
¼ cup chicken stock or water
1 tablespoon dark soy sauce
1 tablespoon thin soy
1 tablespoon black Chinese
vinegar
1 tablespoon dry sherry
1 tablespoon sugar
2 teaspoons sesame oil
1½ tablespoons black beans
About 3 tablespoons cornstarch
for thickening
Oil to stir fry with, a few
teaspoons
2 tablespoons raw cashews,
toasted, or bottled unsalted

Cut the chicken in about 1 to 1½ inch chunks and place in a medium bowl. Toss in the salt and sherry. Mix well. Lightly beat the egg white. Add to the chicken and mix well. Toss in cornstarch. Mix well. Then add the oil and mix again. Allow to sit, covered, at least 30 minutes or as long as overnight.

Bring 2 or 3 quarts of water to a gentle simmer. Put a colander in the sink for draining the chicken. Slide the chicken into the water, stirring gently to separate the pieces. As soon as the outside of the chicken turns white, pour out the water and meat into the colander. This whole procedure is known as velveting and produces some very moist and tender chicken. This procedure may be completed to this point a day or two in advance.

When ready to stir-fry, measure all sauce ingredients into a small glass or measuring cup and set near the range. Mix 3 tablespoons cornstarch to be used for thickening with about an equal amount of water. Stir just before using.

Gather the aromatics and the vegetables near the range. Warm a serving platter in the oven.

Heat a wok or large, heavy skillet until hot. Add about 1 tablespoon cooking oil, swirl to coat the pan. Toss in the whole chiles, stirring and pressing and flipping until they turn nearly black. You may remove them at this point if you wish. Toss in the aromatics, stirring for 15 to 20 seconds. Toss in the bell pepper and scallion and stir-fry for a couple of minutes. Add chicken to the pan, stirring to mix. Then toss in the sauce. Heat the sauce until it bubbles, then add a tablespoon or two of your cornstarch thickening mixture. Stir a bit, judging the thickening and adding a bit more if desired.

The cashews may be used as garnish on the platter, or they may be added to the wok just before the dish is finished. Serve over brown rice. Serves 6.

♨

MARVELOUS MEATLOAF

2 tablespoons margarine	⅓ cup chopped parsley
1 cup finely diced onions	½ teaspoon salt
½ teaspoon rosemary	¼ teaspoon pepper
¼ teaspoon sage	3 pounds frozen ground turkey
1 cup carrots, finely diced	¾ cup unsalted cracker crumbs
1 cup celery, finely diced	⅓ cup skim milk
1 can (4 oz.) mushrooms, sliced	1 egg

In large skillet melt margarine. Add onions and sauté until translucent. Crumble in herbs. Add carrots and celery, sauté until just tender (about 2 minutes). Add mushrooms, cook until liquid evaporates. Stir in parsley, salt, and pepper. Cool. In large bowl combine with remaining ingredients. Shape into 8 x 5 inch loaf pan. Bake 75-90 minutes at 350°. Serve warm or sliced cold. Serves 8.

CHUCK'S CHICKEN & VEGETABLES

8-12 ounces chicken cut into
½-inch chunks
2 tablespoons safflower oil
2-4 cloves garlic, minced
2-4 shallots, minced
½ teaspoon dried oregano (1½
teaspoons if fresh)
½ teaspoon dried basil (1½
teaspoons if fresh)

Fresh ground pepper to taste
1 large onion cut into 1-inch
chunks
1 large green pepper cut into
1-inch chunks
1 pound quartered mushrooms
½-⅔ cup white wine
2-3 tablespoons chopped parsley

Skin, bone, and remove fat and tendons from enough chicken breasts for 2-3 ounces of chicken per serving. Cut into chunks. Add oil to 10-inch sauté pan on medium-high heat. When oil is hot, add garlic, shallots, oregano, basil, and fresh ground pepper. Stir 1-2 minutes. Add chicken chunks, stirring constantly, until all sides have changed color (3-5 minutes). Add onion, green pepper, and mushrooms. Stir 1-2 minutes. Add white wine, scraping the bottom of the pan to loosen any stuck chicken bits. Cook over medium-low heat for about 3 minutes to evaporate alcohol from wine. Cover and cook until vegetables are tender. Sprinkle with parsley just before serving. Serve with brown rice. Serves 4.

❧

HAYDEN'S CHICKEN DELIGHT

4 chicken breasts, skinned
1 egg or 2 egg whites, beaten
1 cup whole wheat bread crumbs
1 tablespoon margarine

1 package spaghetti sauce mix
(tomato)
¼ cup part-skim mozzarella
cheese, grated

Dip chicken in egg and coat with bread crumbs. Brown in margarine. Cook sauce as directed on package. Pour over chicken and bake for 45 minutes at 375°. Sprinkle cheese on each piece of chicken and bake for 10 minutes more. Serves 4.

LEMON CHICKEN

1 fryer (2½-3 pounds), cut up,
    skinned
1 tablespoon grated lemon peel
⅓ cup fresh lemon juice
2 cloves garlic, minced
2 teaspoons dried thyme
1 shallot, finely chopped

½ teaspoon salt
1 teaspoon pepper
1 tablespoon margarine
1 lemon, thinly sliced
½ cup fresh parsley, finely
    chopped

Combine lemon peel, lemon juice, garlic, thyme, shallot, salt, and pepper in a mixing bowl, then pour over chicken pieces placed in a single layer in a shallow baking dish. Marinate in refrigerator 3-4 hours, turning chicken several times. Remove chicken and drain well on paper towels, reserving the marinade. Place chicken in single layer in a shallow 2-quart baking dish. Brush with melted margarine and bake, uncovered, in preheated 425° oven for 25 minutes. Brush with marinade, lower heat to 325°, and bake for another 30-35 minutes or until chicken is brown and thoroughly cooked. Serve surrounded with lemon slices and sprinkled with parsley. Heat and serve marinade separately. Serves 6.

⚜

POLYNESIAN DINNER

¼ cup orange juice
1 can (8 oz.) pineapple chunks,
    undrained
1 tablespoon brown sugar
1 tablespoon soy sauce
1 tablespoon onion flakes

½ green pepper, sliced
2 stalks celery, sliced
1 can (4 oz.) mushrooms, drained
¾ cup cooked meat (chicken,
    lean beef, or lean pork)

Combine all ingredients except meat and simmer for 10 minutes. Add meat and simmer for 5 minutes. Serve over rice. Serves 2.

SUPER LOW CALORIE CHICKEN

2 fryer breasts (about 12 ounces)
3 cups water
2 chicken bouillon cubes
3 tablespoons lemon juice
½ teaspoon dried tarragon leaves
2 bay leaves
1 medium onion, quartered
Pinch of celery leaves

Few sprigs parsley
1 teaspoon cooking oil
½ teaspoon paprika

Lemon Sauce:
1 tablespoon cornstarch
1 tablespoon water
1 teaspoon grated lemon rind

Halve and skin the chicken breasts. Place in saucepan with all the ingredients except cooking oil, paprika, cornstarch, and lemon rind. Bring to boil, reduce heat, and simmer gently until breasts are fork tender, about 30 minutes. Reserve cooking liquid. Place chicken on foil-lined shallow pan, brush lightly with oil mixed with paprika, and place under broiler until chicken is lightly browned. Transfer to platter. Strain cooking liquid and measure 1 cup. Skim off fat. Bring to boil and thicken with cornstarch mixed with water. Stir in grated lemon rind. Garnish chicken with lemon slices and serve with lemon sauce. Serves 4.

⚜

CHICKENBURGERS

2 cups chicken, skinned, cooked,
and minced
1 tablespoon almonds, chopped
½ teaspoon onion, grated
¼ cup dry bread crumbs

2 teaspoons parsley, chopped
1 teaspoon lemon juice
¼ cup milk—skim or low fat
2 tablespoons margarine

Combine all ingredients except margarine. Mix well. Shape mixture into 8 patties. Melt margarine in skillet. Place patties in skillet and sauté until browned on both sides. Serve on toasted buns. Serves 8.

QUICK CHICK SKILLET

3 whole fryer breasts, skinned,
  boned, and cut in 10-12 strips
1 can (1 lb., 4½ oz.) pineapple
  chunks
¾ cup water
2 tablespoons fresh minced onion
1 teaspoon dried leaf tarragon
1 chicken bouillon cube

2 tablespoons soft margarine
1 green pepper, cut in strips
1 cup celery, diagonally sliced
2 tablespoons cornstarch
1 can (4 oz.) pimientos, drained
  and diced
Hot cooked rice

Drain pineapple, combine ½ cup pineapple syrup in a 2-cup measure with ½ cup water, onion, tarragon, and bouillon cube. Heat margarine in large skillet over high heat. Add chicken and cook, stirring constantly, 3 minutes. Add green pepper and celery and cook 2 minutes longer, continuing to stir. Add drained pineapple chunks with syrup mixture. Bring to boil, reduce heat to medium, cover, and cook 4 minutes. Blend together cornstarch and ¼ cup cold water. Stir all at once into skillet and cook, stirring rapidly, until thickened. Add pimiento and serve over hot cooked rice. Serves 6.

ॐ

CHICKEN BREASTS WITH SHERRY

4 chicken breast halves
½ cup buttermilk
3-4 tablespoons flour

Rosemary
1 tablespoon margarine
⅓ cup sherry

Remove skin and fat from chicken breasts. Dip in buttermilk and flour. Add crushed rosemary to taste. Brown quickly in margarine and place in 425° oven for 15-20 minutes, depending on thickness of chicken. Remove from pan and keep warm. Reheat pan on top of stove and add ⅓ cup sherry. Cook and stir at medium high temperature, scraping bottom of pan, until thickened. Pour over chicken breasts. Serve with noodles and fresh asparagus. Serves 4.

CHICKEN BREASTS WITH APRICOTS & AVOCADO

3 whole fryer breasts, split,
  boned, and skinned
½ teaspoon salt
½ teaspoon pepper
¼ teaspoon nutmeg
2 tablespoons margarine
4 green onions, thinly sliced,
  about ¼ cup

¼ cup white wine
1 cup low fat milk
12 fresh apricots, halved
  (preserved or canned apricots
  may be substituted)
2 tablespoons minced parsley
1 ripe avocado
1 tablespoon lemon juice

Sprinkle the chicken with salt, pepper, and nutmeg. Brown the chicken on all sides in melted margarine over medium heat, then remove from pan. Add green onion and brown lightly. Return all the breasts to the pan and add white wine. Cover and simmer 8-10 minutes or until done. Do not overcook. Remove chicken and keep warm. Add the milk to pan juices and stir over high heat until thickened. Add apricots and parsley to warm the fruit. Arrange chicken on a platter. Spoon apricots around and pour sauce over. Slice the avocado, drizzle with lemon, and arrange around the chicken. Serves 6.

⚜

CHICKEN WITH CUMIN & GINGER

3 whole chicken breasts, skinned,
  boned, and cut in half
2 garlic cloves
1 teaspoon ground cumin
2 tablespoons olive oil

½ cup red wine or ¼ cup fruit
  vinegar
1 tablespoon shredded fresh
  ginger

Mix all dry and liquid ingredients to make marinade. Place chicken in shallow bowl with marinade, cover, leaving for 24 hours to 3 days and turning frequently. Heat oil in skillet and sauté until golden brown. Reduce heat, cover, and simmer about 15 minutes. Turn to coat with liquid in pan. Serves 6.

ORIENTAL TURKEY STIR-FRY

1 package (1½ lbs.) fresh turkey
   breast slices, cut in ¼-inch
   strips
1 tablespoon oil
1 bunch (1 pound) bok choy,
   broccoli, snow peas, or any
   desired combination of
   vegetables, sliced
1 can (8 oz.) water chestnuts,
   drained and sliced

1 cup (2 oz.) fresh mushrooms,
   sliced
3 green onions, sliced

Oriental Sauce:
1 cup chicken broth
¼ cup soy sauce
2 tablespoons dry sherry
2 tablespoons cornstarch
¼ teaspoon garlic powder
¼ teaspoon ground ginger

Heat oil in wok or Dutch oven on medium-high for 2-3 minutes. Add turkey. Stir-fry 3-5 minutes until turkey turns white and begins to brown; remove to plate. Add vegetables to wok. Stir-fry 4-5 minutes. Combine sauce ingredients. Pour over vegetables. Add turkey. Heat and stir 2-3 minutes more until sauce is thickened. Serve over rice. Serves 6.

❧

BAKED CHICKEN

4 chicken breasts, skinned
½ cup flour
1¼ teaspoons salt
¼ teaspoon garlic powder
¼ teaspoon basil
1 teaspoon tarragon
¼ teaspoon rosemary
¼ teaspoon paprika

2 tablespoons oil

Sauce:
1 cup mushrooms, sliced
¼ cup lemon juice
1 teaspoon onion, minced
1 clove garlic, mashed
½ cup white wine

Mix dry ingredients in paper bag. Shake chicken in bag then brown in oil. Drain and place in baking dish. Combine sauce ingredients and brush over chicken. Bake at 375° for 1 hour, basting often. Serves 4.

CHICKEN BREASTS WITH CURRIED FRUIT

2 tablespoons margarine
4 half chicken breasts, skinned and boned
1 teaspoon curry powder
2 tablespoons dry vermouth or dry white wine
½ teaspoon salt (optional)

½ cup Oregon prunes, pitted
2 cups grapes, peaches, pears, and pineapple, diced
2 tablespoons brown sugar
1 tablespoon toasted slivered almonds

In large heavy skillet, melt margarine over medium heat. Add chicken breasts. Sauté until light brown on both sides. While browning chicken, stir curry powder into margarine. Add vermouth or wine, salt, and prunes. Cover and simmer over low heat 5-7 minutes. To test doneness, press finger into thickest part of chicken breast; meat should spring back. Place chicken breasts on a plate and cover with skillet lid to keep warm. Add fruit and brown sugar to pan juices and bring to a boil. Cook until syrupy. Place chicken breasts on platter or individual plates. Pour sauce over. Top with toasted almonds. Serves 4.

❧

CHICKEN & PRUNES

4 chicken breast halves, skinned and fat removed (with wings attached)
Ground pepper to taste
2 teaspoons crushed cumin seed

1 teaspoon paprika
2 garlic cloves, crushed
8 ounces prunes, pitted
2 cups water
1 medium onion

Place chicken in large heavy casserole. Sprinkle pepper, cumin, paprika, and garlic over chicken; set aside for 30 minutes. Soak prunes in water to plump. Thinly slice onion and separate into rings. Arrange over and around chicken with prunes and about 1 cup of the prune water. Cover and bake in a preheated 350° oven, adding more prune water if needed until chicken is tender—about 1 hour. Serves 4.

CHICKEN FLORENTINE

2 whole fryer breasts, boned,
  halved, and skinned
1 teaspoon salt
¼ cup flour
1 tablespoon oil
1 package (10 oz.) frozen chopped
  spinach

1 ounce grated Parmesan cheese
1 ounce part-skim mozzarella
  cheese, sliced
⅓ cup white wine
Juice of ½ lemon
½ cup chicken broth

Dredge the chicken in salted flour. Sauté in vegetable oil 10 minutes on each side. Cook and drain spinach and set aside. Place chicken in heavy metal baking dish. Cover each breast with spinach. Sprinkle Parmesan cheese over spinach. Cover with sliced mozzarella. Bake at 350° for 35 minutes. Remove chicken to heated platter and keep warm. To make sauce add wine and lemon juice to pan. Simmer and scrape until liquid is half gone. Add chicken broth, stir, and simmer 2 minutes. Pour sauce over chicken or serve separately. Serves 4.

❧

CHICKEN CREOLE

2½ to 3 pounds fryer parts,
  skinned
½ teaspoon salt
½ teaspoon paprika
1 medium onion, sliced
1 medium green pepper, cut in
  strips

½ cup celery, diced
1 can (16 oz.) tomatoes
1 can (3 or 4 oz.) mushrooms
2 tablespoons parsley, chopped

Sprinkle chicken with ¼ teaspoon each of salt and paprika. Brown in nonstick or lightly oiled skillet. Remove chicken from pan. Put in remaining ingredients. Bring to boil, cover, and cook 10 minutes. Add chicken. Cover; reduce heat and simmer 40 minutes. Turn into serving dish; sprinkle with parsley. Serves 6.

TURKEY POLYNESIAN

1-1½ pounds turkey breast,
skinned, boned, and cut into
small cubes
1 tablespoon cornstarch
1 teaspoon salt
2 teaspoons water
1 teaspoon soy sauce
1 cup onion, sliced

2 tablespoons oil
1 cup celery, diagonally sliced
1 can water chestnuts, drained
and sliced
1 cup canned pineapple in own
juice, chunks or tidbits
¼ cup pineapple juice
Hot cooked rice

Combine cornstarch, salt, water, and soy sauce. Dredge turkey cubes in cornstarch mixture. Sauté onion in 1 tablespoon oil. Add celery and water chestnuts; cook 2 minutes. Remove vegetables form pan. Sauté turkey in remaining 1 tablespoon oil until brown. Add vegetables, pineapple, and pineapple juice. Simmer 10 minutes. Serve hot with rice. Serves 6.

⚜

TURKEY (CHICKEN) STIR-FRY

1 cup chopped skinned turkey or
chicken (cooked or raw)
⅛ cup sherry
⅛ cup dark corn syrup
⅛ cup low-salt soy sauce
1 package Near East frozen
vegetables

2 tablespoons sliced almonds or
cashews
Non-stick cooking spray
1 cup cooked pasta or rice

Skin chicken or turkey. Marinate in liquid mixture for 1-2 hours. Spray wok or fry pan with cooking spray. Stir-fry poultry (raw poultry 2 minutes or cooked poultry 1 minute), set aside. Stir in frozen vegetables, steam with lid on 2-3 minutes; add poultry and nuts. Serve over pasta or rice. Serves 4.

BAKED CHICKEN WITH MUSHROOMS & ONIONS

1 frying chicken (2½-3 pounds),
   cut up, skinned, washed, and
   patted dry
2 cups medium white sauce
½ cup green onions, chopped
½ cup mushrooms, sliced
Pepper and poultry seasoning to
   taste

White Sauce:
3 tablespoons cornstarch
2 cups low fat milk
2 tablespoons margarine
½ teaspoon salt
½ teaspoon pepper

Pepper and season chicken and arrange in baking dish. Cover and bake for 30 minutes at 275°.

Mix cornstarch and milk until smooth, add margarine, salt, and pepper and bring to boil over medium heat, stirring constantly. Boil 1 minute. Add onions, mushrooms, and stock from chicken. Blend well and pour over chicken and bake additional 15 minutes. Serves 6.

❧

CHICKEN CARUSO

1 slice Canadian bacon, finely cut
½ cup onion, minced
½ cup green pepper, minced
1½ cups cooked skinned chicken,
   cut up
2 tablespoons part-skim
   mozzarella cheese, grated

2 tablespoons (2 oz. jar) pimiento,
   cut up
1 cup cooked peas
⅛ teaspoon each salt and pepper
3 cups hot drained boiled
   macaroni (1½ cups uncooked)
Parsley

In medium skillet, sauté bacon until lightly browned and crisp. Stir in onion and green pepper, cook until almost tender. Stir in chicken, cheese, pimiento, and peas. Season with salt and pepper. Mix in cooked macaroni. Cover and keep warm over very low heat until ready to serve. Garnish with parsley. Serves 4.

CHICKEN SUKIYAKI

3 chicken breasts, skinned and
  boned
1 small onion
1 cup water chestnuts
1 cup bamboo shoots
⅔ cup celery
⅔ cup mushrooms
1½ cups fresh spinach
⅔ cup red sweet peppers

1 can shiritake noodles
Optional: any vegetable can be
  used

Sauce:
⅓ cup soy sauce
⅔ cup water
⅔ cup white wine

Slice all ingredients on diagonal. Use large teflon fry pan, wok, or cast iron skillet with non-stick spray. Sauté on medium-high temperature onion slices, chicken slices, then each vegetable according to density. Pour sauce over all. Cook 5-6 minutes on medium temperature. Serve with rice. Serves 6.

♣

LEMONY CHICKEN BREASTS

4 chicken breasts, skinned, all
  visible fat removed
Juice of 2 lemons

1 clove garlic, minced
1 tablespoon soy sauce
4 tablespoons honey

Marinate chicken in combined seasonings at least 1 hour. Bake in shallow baking dish for about 1½ hours at 325°, basting frequently. Time of cooking depends on the size of the chicken breasts. Serves 4.

CRISPY OVEN-FRIED LEMON CHICKEN

1 fryer, cut into serving pieces
   and skinned
½ teaspoon salt
½ small onion, diced
½ teaspoon thyme, crushed
½ teaspoon marjoram, crushed

2 teaspoons grated lemon peel
⅓ cup fresh lemon juice
½ cup water
Lemon quarters
Paprika
Snipped parsley

Sprinkle chicken pieces with salt, rubbing well into flesh. Place in shallow baking pan. Combine seasonings, lemon peel and juice, and water; pour over chicken. Bake uncovered at 350° about 30 minutes. Turn chicken and continue to bake, basting with pan drippings once or twice, until chicken is done, about 30 minutes. Dust one cut side of each lemon quarter with paprika; sprinkle other cut side with finely snipped parsley. Garnish serving platter with lemon quarters so guests can squeeze juice over for additional tang. Serves 3-4.

🌿

POULTRY IN A POCKET-TO-GO

1 teaspoon margarine
½ teaspoon prepared mustard
Dash onion powder
1 pita bread (1 ounce) cut in half
   crosswise to form 2 pockets
1 ounce skinned and boned
   cooked chicken, chilled and
   sliced

4 lettuce leaves
½ medium tomato, sliced
¼ cup each cucumber slices and
   carrot sticks

In a cup blend margarine with mustard and onion powder; spread inside of each pita pocket with half of the mustard butter, then stuff 1 ounce chicken into each. Place cut ends of pita together and wrap sandwich in plastic wrap; wrap vegetables individually in plastic wrap or resealable plastic bags. Makes 1 serving.

CHESTNUT DRESSING
(For 12-lb. Turkey)

Oil (just enough to sauté)
½ cup onion
1 cup celery, chopped
1 cup raisins
4 cups apples, pared, cored, and
    chopped
6 cups whole wheat bread
    crumbs

4 cups chestnuts, coarsely
    chopped
1 teaspoon salt
1 teaspoon cinnamon
¼ teaspoon nutmeg

Sauté onion and celery in oil until tender. In large bowl, with fork, toss remaining ingredients with onion and celery until combined.

Note: If you line the inside of the turkey with cheesecloth before stuffing, the dressing will be easier to remove.

FISH & SHELLFISH

Fish and shellfish are the best choice among animal protein foods because they are very low in fat. Eat some at least twice a week instead of meat. Remember, fresh or frozen is preferable to smoked or otherwise cured.

Rapid cooking is essential to retaining the moist tenderness of fish and shellfish. And they can be used frozen in most recipes. The simpler the recipe, the more the flavor and texture will come through.

BAKED HALIBUT

1 yellow onion, sliced
1 lemon, sliced
White wine to cover ½ inch of
   baking dish

1½ pounds halibut
½ cup celery, chopped
⅛ teaspoon pepper
¾ cup Italian bread crumbs

Place onions on bottom of baking dish with lemon slices on top. Pour ½ inch of white wine over onions and lemons. Place halibut in dish and sprinkle with celery and pepper. Cover with bread crumbs. Bake fish at 350° until flaky. Serves 4.

🌿

BAKED TROUT IN WINE

6 rainbow trout
2 tablespoons lemon juice
1 teaspoon salt
Pepper to taste
1 cup dry white wine
2 tablespoons parsley, chopped
¼ cup green onions, sliced

2 tablespoons fine dry bread
   crumbs
2 tablespoons margarine, melted
Fresh dill (dried dill weed may be
   substituted)
6 fresh lemon slices

Preheat oven to 400°. Wash and dry trout. Brush insides of fish with lemon juice and sprinkle with salt and pepper. Arrange trout in shallow baking dish and brush with remaining lemon juice. Pour wine into bottom of dish. Sprinkle fish evenly with parsley and onions. Sprinkle with bread crumbs lightly and spoon melted margarine over each piece of fish. Bake uncovered for 25 minutes. Garnish with dill and lemon slices. Serves 6.

ARLENE'S MOTHER'S SOLE

2 tablespoons oil
   (optional)
6 green onions with tops, minced
½ pound mushrooms, slivered
4 large fillets of sole
⅛ teaspoon soy sauce
1 small can mandarin oranges,
   drained

¼ cup orange juice
½ cup white wine
3 tablespoons curaçao liqueur
¼ teaspoon salt
Pepper to taste
2 tablespoons parsley, minced

Place 1 tablespoon oil in bottom of baking dish and cover with 1 table-spoon of the onions and half of the slivered mushrooms. Place 2 fish fillets on top. Sprinkle with half of the soy sauce, oranges, juice, wine, and liqueur. Place remaining fish on top. Add rest of onions, mushrooms, juice, seasonings, and oranges. Place in preheated 350° oven for about 45 minutes or until the top is slightly brown. Garnish with parsley. Serves 4.

❧

STIR-FRIED FISH DINNER

1 tablespoon oil
2 tablespoons water
1 tablespoon onion, chopped
1 tablespoon garlic, minced
1 tablespoon ginger, grated
1 green pepper, cubed
2 tomatoes, cubed

½ cup vegetables, chopped
   (broccoli, zucchini, carrots,
   etc.)
⅓-½ cup mushrooms, sliced
1 pound fresh fish (trout, salmon
   fillets, or other)
¼ cup sherry (optional)

Heat the oil and water in a non-stick fry pan at medium heat (300°). Add seasonings and vegetables, gently stirring for 5 minutes. Add the fish and cook for about 3-5 minutes per side (or until done); the sherry may be added at this time. Garnish with fresh parsley. Serves 2-4.

PORTUGUESE FISHERMAN STEW

2 pounds white fish fillets, fresh
   or frozen
1 tablespoon margarine
1 cup onion, chopped
1 clove garlic, crushed
2 cans (1 lb. each) tomatoes,
   undrained, cut up
3 cups water

1 teaspoon leaf basil
1 teaspoon leaf thyme
¼ teaspoon crushed red pepper
1 teaspoon salt
4 cups pumpkin or winter squash,
   cut into 1-inch cubes
2 ears corn, cut crosswise into
   1-inch pieces

Thaw fish if frozen. Cut fish into 1-inch cubes. In a large saucepan melt margarine. Add onion and garlic and cook until vegetables are tender. Add tomatoes, water, basil, thyme, red pepper, salt, pumpkin, and corn. Cover and bring to a boil; simmer for 10-15 minutes or until pumpkin and corn are done. Add fish and continue to cook for 5-10 minutes or until fish flakes easily when tested with a fork. Makes 12 cups.

⚜

TUNA LOAF

1 can water-packed tuna, drained
½ yellow onion, minced
2 teaspoons lemon juice
1 egg, beaten, or 2 egg whites
Skim milk, enough to moisten

Pepper to taste
¼ cup mushrooms, chopped
¼ cup celery, chopped
1 slice whole wheat bread

Mix all of the ingredients in a bowl, except bread. Rinse bread under water and squeeze out water. Add moistened bread to mixture. Place evenly in greased loaf pan. Cook for 40-45 minutes at 350° until brown. Slice and serve warm. Serves 2-3.

SALMON-STUFFED POTATOES

6 large potatoes, baked
1½ cups mushrooms, chopped
2 tablespoons margarine
1 tablespoon parsley, chopped

1 can (16 oz.) red salmon, drained
⅔ cup low fat milk
1 medium onion, chopped

Slice off tops of potatoes and scoop out insides. Sauté mushrooms in margarine until moisture is evaporated. Add parsley. Divide mushroom mixture among potato shells. Whip salmon, potato centers, and milk until smooth. Season to taste. Spoon mixture into potato shells; reheat in a 350° oven. If desired, garnish with fluted mushrooms. Serves 6.

🍃

STUFFED FLOUNDER FILLETS

2 teaspoons oil
1 cup mushrooms, chopped
½ cup scallions, chopped
1 garlic clove, minced
¼ teaspoon salt
⅛ teaspoon each pepper and
   ground thyme

1 tablespoon plus 1½ teaspoons
   plain dried bread crumbs
2 flounder fillets, 5 ounces each
1 teaspoon each lemon juice and
   chopped parsley

Preheat oven to 400°. In small skillet, heat 1 teaspoon oil; add vegetables and seasonings and sauté 5 minutes. Stir in crumbs. Sprinkle fillets with lemon juice and spoon half of stuffing onto each; roll fillets to enclose filling. Place seam-side down in shallow 1 quart casserole and sprinkle each roll with remaining oil. Bake 15 minutes and sprinkle with parsley. Serves 2.

NORTHWEST CIOPPINO

1½ pounds ling cod, perch, red
   snapper (or other rockfish)
2 cups onion, sliced
2 cloves garlic, finely minced
2 tablespoons vegetable oil
3½ cups (no. 2½ can) tomatoes,
   undrained
1 can (8 oz.) tomato sauce

1 cup water
¼ cup parsley, chopped
1 teaspoon salt
1 teaspoon basil
½ teaspoon oregano
¼ teaspoon pepper
1 dozen clams, washed, in shell
1 cup shrimp, cooked and peeled

Cut fish into 1½-inch chunks. Cook onion and garlic in oil until onion is tender but not brown. Add tomatoes, tomato sauce, water, parsley, salt, basil, oregano, and pepper. Cover. Simmer gently about 30 minutes. Add fish chunks and clams; cover and simmer 10 minutes or less until fish flakes with fork. Add precooked shrimp. Serves 6.

✣

BAKED ORANGE ROUGHY

½ cup celery, chopped
1½ pounds Orange Roughy
½ teaspoon salt
¼ teaspoon rosemary

¼ teaspoon paprika
1 medium tomato, sliced
½ cup scallions, chopped
¼ cup white wine

Cover bottom of a baking dish with celery. Arrange the fish on celery, overlapping edges if needed. Sprinkle with spices, arrange tomato slices over fish and sprinkle with scallions. Pour wine over top and bake at 350° for 25 minutes. Serves 4.

FILLET OF SOLE WITH GARLIC & SPINACH

25 medium cloves garlic (about
  1½ heads), baked
16 large spinach leaves
8 medium fillets of sole
Salt and white pepper
Juice of 1 lemon

Fish Stock:
1 tablespoon soft margarine
1 medium onion, sliced

1-1½ pounds fish bones, cut into
  pieces or reserved bones from
  8 medium fillets of sole
1 quart water
10 whole peppercorns
Bouquet garni made from
  parsley, thyme, and bay leaf

To make stock, place margarine in a large pot and cook onion over medium heat until soft but not browned, about 8-10 minutes. Add fish bones, water, peppercorns, and bouquet garni and bring to a boil. Skim and simmer, uncovered, for 20 minutes. Strain and set aside.

Squeeze baked garlic cloves out of their skins into a bowl. Mash with a fork to make a spreadable puree, and set aside. In a large pot, blanch spinach leaves in enough water to cover by holding stem end of each leaf and dipping it into rapidly boiling water for 1 minute. Remove, rinse with cold water, and drain on paper towels. Place fillets of sole on a work surface, skin side up, and make several shallow slashes. Spread each fillet evenly with pureed garlic and season with salt and pepper. Place a spinach leaf over each fillet, folding edges inward so spinach is the same width as the sole and covers garlic puree completely. Sprinkle with a little lemon juice and more salt and pepper.

Roll each fillet from one narrow end to the other. Place a leaf of spinach, inside up, on work surface, and position the rolled fillet inside it. Fold edges of spinach up and over sides of fillet and roll evenly towards the other end so fish is covered completely. Secure rolls with toothpicks, if necessary. In a large shallow pan, bring fish stock to a boil. Immediately reduce to simmer. Never allow stock to boil once fish has been added. Poach fish rolls in stock for 5-7 minutes, carefully roll them over and poach another 5-7 minutes. Lift from poaching liquid with a slotted spoon, allow to drain, and serve immediately. Serves 8.

FILLET OF FISH FLORENTINE

2 pounds red snapper or other
white fish cut into serving size
4 peppercorns
½ bay leaf
2 teaspoons lemon juice
½ cup bread crumbs

Florentine Sauce:
1 package frozen chopped
spinach

2 tablespoons margarine
1 tablespoon onion, finely
chopped
2 tablespoons flour
1 cup skim milk
½ teaspoon each salt and pepper
¼ teaspoon each, oregano and
thyme (optional)

Place fish fillets in skillet. Cover with boiling water. Season with pepper-corns, bay leaf, and lemon juice. Simmer about 10 minutes or until ten-der. Remove fish with slotted spoon and place in bottom of oven-proof platter. Cook spinach according to package directions and drain well. Melt margarine in a skillet. Add onion and cook until golden. Stir in flour until blended. Add milk slowly and stir until sauce is smooth and thick-ened slightly. Add drained, cooked spinach. Season with salt and pepper. Pour spinach in sauce over poached fish. Sprinkle bread crumbs on top. Place under broiler to heat through until sauce is glazed. Serve immedi-ately. Serves 6.

⚓

PERCH PIQUANT

2 pounds fillets of perch, snapper,
or other rockfish, cut into
serving pieces

1 teaspoon salt
1 tablespoon prepared mustard
⅛ teaspoon curry powder

Sprinkle fillets with salt. Add curry to mustard and spread evenly over lean side of fish. Place in a lightly greased pan and bake covered in a 400° oven for 8-10 minutes depending on thickness of the fillets. Serves 5-6.

LINGUINE WITH CLAM SAUCE

1 pound linguine noodles, cooked and drained (fettuccine noodles are a great substitute)

Sauce:

36 small clams, opened, or 2 cans minced clams with juice

2 tablespoons oil

3 cloves garlic, chopped

½ cup dry white wine

¼ cup chopped parsley

¼ teaspoon each oregano, basil, pepper

¼ cup Parmesan cheese, grated

Remove the clams from shells, reserving the juice, or drain clams from cans, saving the juice. In a skillet, heat oil and sauté garlic until golden. Add clams and stir until clams are just cooked, about 5 minutes. Add clam liquor plus remaining ingredients. Simmer 5 minutes. Place hot cooked noodles on serving plates, top with clam sauce, and sprinkle with Parmesan cheese. Serves 6.

BANANA PRAWN CURRY

6 medium onions, thinly sliced

2 tablespoons margarine

2-3 teaspoons curry powder

1 cup low fat milk

1 cube chicken bouillon

½ cup hot water

2 medium bananas, sliced

1½ pounds prawns, cooked and cleaned

Cook onions over low heat in margarine until clear and golden. Add curry powder and milk. Dissolve bouillon cube in hot water. Add to onions and cook over medium heat 10 minutes. Add bananas and cook 10 minutes longer, stirring occasionally. Add prawns and cook over low heat just until shrimp are heated through. Serve over hot rice. Accompany with condiments such as chutney. Serves 4.

SWEET & SOUR SCALLOPS

1½ pounds bay scallops
1 cup white wine for poaching
4 peppercorns or ½ teaspoon
    cracked black pepper
½ pound snow peas, ends
    trimmed
1 can (8 oz.) water chestnuts,
    sliced
2 small red peppers, seeded and
    cut into 1-inch squares
4 cups cooked brown rice
Optional: oranges and bananas,
    sliced

Sweet and Sour Sauce:
⅓ cup ketchup
¼ cup cider vinegar
¼ cup apple juice
½ teaspoon sugar
2 teaspoons soy sauce
½ cup water
1½ tablespoons cornstarch

Pour wine in a large skillet. Add black pepper. Bring to a simmer; poach scallops for about 3 minutes. At this point, the scallops should not be fully cooked. Drain wine and return scallops to skillet. Set aside. Plunge snow peas into a saucepan of boiling water and blanch for 4 minutes. Drain. Similarly blanch red pepper.

Combine all sauce ingredients except water and cornstarch in a small saucepan and bring to a slow boil. Mix cornstarch into water and add slowly to boiling sauce, stirring constantly. Continue to cook over medium heat, stirring, until sauce is thickened, about 7 minutes.

Add snow peas, peppers, and water chestnuts to skillet with scallops. Add sauce and stir over low heat for 2 or 3 minutes, coating vegetables and scallops with sauce. Remove from heat. (May be frozen.) Serve over rice with sliced fruit. Serves 8.

CASSEROLES

Casseroles share many virtues with salads. Because they are made with a variety of ingredients, casseroles can be a good source of fiber (whole grains, beans) and of vitamin A and C (green leafy and yellow vegetables) in addition to all other nutrients. Be careful not to add excessive amounts of nuts, seeds, or cheeses to them.

The principal ingredients of casseroles are pasta, potatoes, and rice—main staples in much of the world. These foods do not require much energy to produce. They are both economical and ecologically sound.

In a diet to reduce the risk of cancer, beef, pork, lamb, or ham simply accompany vegetables, pasta, rice, or other grains. We have used only small amounts of meat in those casseroles calling for meat. Try to limit red meat dishes to two or three a week; it is a good way to limit fat in your diet.

TUNA & GREEN BEAN CASSEROLE

2 tablespoons onion, minced
1 tablespoon oil
2 tablespoons flour
1 cup skim milk
¼ cup chicken bouillon
1 tablespoon prepared mustard
2 cups green beans, cooked

1 hard-boiled egg, chopped
1 can (7 oz.) water-packed tuna,
   drained and flaked
1 tablespoon parsley, minced
½ teaspoon dried tarragon
Pepper
¼ cup cornflakes, dry

Cook onions in oil until wilted. Add flour, milk, and bouillon. Stir constantly until thickened. Add mustard, beans, egg, tuna, parsley, and tarragon. Taste; add pepper if needed. Put in 1-quart casserole dish and sprinkle with cornflakes. Bake at 400° for about 20 minutes. Serves 4.

❧

SEAFOOD CASSEROLE

1 medium onion, chopped
2 teaspoons margarine
2 teaspoons paprika
¼ teaspoon oregano
¼ teaspoon garlic powder
2 cups plain bread crumbs

1 can (6½ oz.) whole baby clams
2 cups skim milk
½ pound small shrimp
1 tablespoon parsley
¼ cup grated part-skim
   mozzarella cheese

In large pan sauté onion in margarine. Add paprika, oregano, and garlic powder. Remove from heat. Add bread crumbs, clams with broth, milk, shrimp, parsley, and ¼ cup of the cheese. Let rest for 5-10 minutes. Add more milk or crumbs, if needed, to make a medium thickness. Put everything in lightly oiled oven dish and top with remaining ¼ cup cheese and paprika. Bake at 325° for 30 minutes. Serves 4.

TURKEY CURRY CASSEROLE

Water for sautéing
2 large onions, chopped
½ teaspoon ground ginger
⅛ teaspoon cinnamon
3 tablespoons curry powder
½ cup lemon juice
3½ cups chicken stock

Freshly ground black pepper
2 pounds boneless, skinless turkey
   breast, cut into 1 inch cubes
1½ cups uncooked brown rice
1 package (10 oz.) frozen peas,
   cooked
¼ cup chopped cashews

Heat a shallow layer of water in a large nonstick saucepan. Add onions, ginger, cinnamon, and curry powder. Cook over low heat for about 10 minutes, stirring to coat onions with spices. Add lemon juice, stock, and freshly ground pepper. Bring to a boil. Add turkey and rice. Simmer, covered, for about 45 minutes or until liquid is evaporated and turkey is cooked. Add cooked peas and cashews and stir to combine. To freeze, divide into 10 individual freezer containers. To heat from frozen, cook at 375° for 50 minutes or until hot. May serve with a side dish of plain low fat yogurt mixed with chopped cucumber and scallions. Serves 10.

⚜

VEGETARIAN CHILI CASSEROLE

3 cans (28 oz. each) tomato sauce
1 can (28 oz.) whole pack
   tomatoes
3 cans (15 oz. each) Great
   Northern beans, drained
2 cans (27 oz. each) dark red
   kidney beans, drained

1 cup chopped onion
1 cup chopped green pepper
1 cup chopped zucchini
1 cup bean sprouts
1 cup chopped red cabbage
Chili pepper to taste

Put all ingredients in large pot and mix. Be sure tomato sauce covers everything. Simmer on top of stove for 1 hour. Serve over a bed of brown rice. Serves 10.

ELK WITH FRESH BROCCOLI

½ pound elk or lean beef
1 tablespoon sherry or wine
1 tablespoon soy sauce
Dash of pepper
½ onion, sliced thin
1 clove garlic
2 slices ginger root
1 medium carrot, sliced
1½ pounds fresh broccoli (use stems and florets), cut in small pieces

¼ teaspoon salt
3 tablespoons stock or bouillon
½ tablespoon oil
1 tablespoon cornstarch
2 tablespoons water
2 tablespoons oyster sauce (found in Oriental section of grocery stores)

Thinly cut meat across the grain. Marinate with wine, soy sauce, and pepper. Spray skillet with non-stick cooking spray. Heat and add onions, garlic, ginger root. Cook lightly and add carrots and broccoli. Cook until broccoli is a bright green color. Add salt, and stock or bouillon. Remove vegetables and put in a separate bowl. Put oil in skillet. When hot, add meat. Stir-fry meat for 1 minute, lightly tossing as it cooks. Add vegetable mixture and stir-fry for 1½ minutes. Dissolve cornstarch in water. Add to mixture with oyster sauce and heat until thickened. Serve hot. May be served over cooked rice. Serves 4-6.

♣

ALPINE RICE

1½ cups long-grain brown rice, cooked and hot
2 tablespoons Parmesan cheese, grated

2 tablespoons part-skim mozzarella cheese, grated
½ cup skim milk, hot
Pepper to taste

Mix rice and cheeses gently together. Pour hot milk over mixture and toss. Pepper to taste. Serve immediately as side dish or main entree. Serves 4-6.

LOUISIANA CHICKEN CASSEROLE

1 egg and 2 egg whites
1 cup low fat milk
1 cup flour, unsifted
1½ teaspoons salt
Dash of Tabasco pepper sauce
2 cups chicken, skinned, cooked,
   and diced

½ cup pimiento, chopped
¼ cup parsley, chopped
1 tablespoon margarine, melted
1 tablespoon onion, grated
¼ teaspoon dried thyme

Combine eggs, milk, flour, salt, and Tabasco sauce. Beat until well blended. Stir in remaining ingredients and turn into lightly greased 1½ quart casserole. Bake at 350° for 40 minutes or until custard is set. Serve with additional Tabasco sauce. Serves 4.

⚜

CHILI FOR A CROWD

4 pounds ground turkey
6 onions, chopped
4 green peppers, chopped
4-6 tablespoons chili powder
1½ tablespoons salt
1-3 teaspoons cayenne pepper

4 bay leaves
5 cans (16 oz. each) tomatoes,
   cut up
5 cans (30 oz. each) chili beans
1 cup red wine

Brown meat, onions, and green peppers. Add 4 tablespoons chili powder, salt, 1 teaspoon cayenne, and bay leaves. Cook over medium low heat for 30 minutes. Add cut-up tomatoes, chili beans, and wine. Simmer, covered, for at least 2 hours. Add more chili powder and cayenne as needed for desired spiciness. This freezes well, so freeze leftovers in meal-sized portions. Serves 20.

HEALTHY MEATLOAF

1 pound extra lean ground beef
¾ cup oatmeal
1 small onion, finely diced
1 stalk celery, finely diced
1 carrot, finely grated
½ cup plain low fat yogurt
2 tablespoons fresh parsley,
   chopped
2 tablespoons chili sauce

½ teaspoon thyme
½ teaspoon oregano
¼ teaspoon pepper

Tomato Glaze:
½ cup tomato sauce
1 tablespoon Dijon mustard
1 tablespoon brown sugar
¼ teaspoon nutmeg

Combine all ingredients; mix well. Mound in metal pie tin. Top with tomato glaze. Bake in 350° oven for 45-55 minutes. Serves 4-6.

ꬉ

BLACK BEANS & RICE

1 pound dried black beans,
   washed and drained
6 cups water
2 bay leaves
½ teaspoon salt
¼ teaspoon black pepper
4 ounces lean ham or turkey
   ham, chopped

1 cup onion, chopped
1 green pepper, chopped
1 garlic clove, crushed
2 tablespoons olive oil
4 cups cooked rice
Raw sweet onion rings

Cover beans with water and bring to a boil for 2 minutes. Cover pan and let stand for 1 hour. Pour off the water and add 6 cups of fresh water, bay leaves, salt, pepper, and ham. Bring to a boil. Reduce heat and simmer covered for 2 hours, adding more water if necessary.

After the beans have cooked, sauté the chopped onion, green pepper, and garlic in olive oil. Add to the cooked beans. Serve over ¾ cup hot rice and garnish with raw sweet onion rings. Serves 8.

ZUCCHINI RICE CASSEROLE

3 cups zucchini, quartered and sliced
3 cups cooked rice (1 cup uncooked)
¼ cup low fat mozzarella cheese, shredded
1 stalk celery, chopped

1 egg and 2 egg whites, beaten
1 cup onion, finely chopped
¼ teaspoon pepper
Dash of salt
Grated peel and juice of 1 lemon
1 can cream of mushroom soup

Mix ingredients and bake at 350° for 40 minutes. Serves 8.

⚜

FRONTIER HAZELNUT VEGETABLE PIE

1 cup fresh broccoli, chopped*
1 cup fresh cauliflower, sliced*
2 cups fresh spinach, chopped*
1 small onion, diced

*Ten-ounce packages of frozen, chopped broccoli, cauliflower, and spinach may be substituted for fresh. Thaw and drain well. Do not pre-cook.

½ green pepper, diced
¼ cup low fat cheddar cheese, grated
2 tablespoons coarsely chopped hazelnuts, preferably roasted
1½ cups low fat milk
1 cup baking mix
2 eggs or 1 egg and two whites
1 teaspoon salt
Pinch of garlic powder
½ teaspoon pepper

Cook broccoli and cauliflower until almost tender (about 5 minutes). Drain well. Mix broccoli, cauliflower, spinach, onion, green pepper, and cheese and put into a well-greased 10-inch pie plate. Top with hazelnuts. Beat together the milk, baking mix, eggs, garlic salt, and pepper, pour over hazelnuts and vegetables. Bake at 400° for 35-40 minutes; let pie stand 5 minutes before cutting. Serves 6.

HERBED BARLEY

½ cup chopped onion
2 teaspoons safflower oil
⅓ cup chopped green pepper
3 cups chicken broth
1 cup pearl barley

¼ teaspoon each thyme, sage, and marjoram
⅛ teaspoon each salt and black pepper
Pinch of turmeric (optional)

In a medium-sized nonstick saucepan, sauté onion in oil until translucent, about 3 minutes. Add green pepper and cook for 3 minutes more. Add chicken broth and bring to a boil. Add barley and spices. Lower heat and simmer, covered, for about 45 minutes, until just tender. Serves 4.

❧

VEGETABLE CASSEROLE

1½ cups long-grain brown rice, uncooked
2 large tomatoes, sliced
1 zucchini, sliced into ½-inch pieces
1 medium eggplant, peeled and sliced thinly
1 medium yellow onion, chopped

½ cup Italian breadcrumbs
2 eggs or 1 egg and 2 egg whites
½ teaspoon dried oregano
Pepper to taste
¾ pound mushrooms, sliced
2 tablespoons part-skim mozzarella
2 tablespoons Parmesan cheese, grated

Cook rice and spread evenly on bottom of 9 x 11 inch baking dish. Place tomato slices over rice, then layer zucchini slices. Boil eggplant until soft (3-5 minutes), drain, and puree in processor. Add onions, breadcrumbs, eggs, oregano, and pepper to eggplant. Process until smooth. Spread mixture on top of zucchini. Cover eggplant layer with mushrooms. Mix together cheeses and sprinkle over the top. Bake at 350° for about 45 minutes. Serves 6.

BROCCOLI WITH RICE

1 onion, chopped
1 rib celery, chopped
1 tablespoon margarine
1 package chopped frozen
    broccoli or 1½ cups chopped
    fresh broccoli

1 can cream of celery soup (use a
    low-sodium soup if available)
2 cups cooked brown rice
2 drops Tabasco sauce
Bread crumbs
¼ cup Parmesan cheese, grated

Preheat oven to 350°. In large skillet, sauté the onions and celery in margarine until clear. Cook broccoli until barely tender and drain well. Mix broccoli with soup and cheese. Add to celery and onions. Stir in rice and Tabasco sauce and mix well. Pour into a casserole and top with bread crumbs. Bake for about 20 minutes, until bubbly. Serves 3 as a main dish; serves 6 as a side dish.

Options:
1. Add 1 can water chestnuts.
2. Use other grains, such as barley or whole wheat berries, in combination with the brown rice.

❧

LEMON DILL RICE

1 large onion, finely chopped
2 cups long-grain white or brown
    rice
1 tablespoon margarine

4 cups water
1 teaspoon salt
2 tablespoons dill
¼ cup fresh lemon juice

Preheat oven to 325°. Brown the onion and rice in margarine. Add the water, seasonings, and lemon juice. Bring to a boil, then transfer to a 3-quart casserole. Bake for 1 hour. Serves 8.

BROCCOLI-CORN CASSEROLE

1 package (10 oz.) frozen chopped
   broccoli, thawed (fresh may be
   used)
1 can (17 oz.) cream-style corn
½ onion, chopped
¼ cup saltine crackers, crushed
1 egg, well-beaten, or 2 egg
   whites

Dash pepper

Topping:
2 tablespoons margarine, melted
2 tablespoons saltine crackers,
   crushed

Mix the main ingredients. Pour into 1½ quart casserole. Sprinkle topping over all. Bake uncovered at 350° for 1 hour. Serves 6.

❧

STIR-FRIED MUSHROOMS & TOFU

1 tablespoon margarine
½ pound mushrooms, fresh and
   cut into quarters
¼ cup chopped onions
½ can water chestnuts, cut into
   small pieces

½ can bamboo shoots, cut into
   small pieces
Dash of seasoned salt
Tofu—about a quarter to a half
   tub will do
2½ tablespoons oyster sauce

Heat wok or frying pan to medium-high temperature. Melt margarine in the pan. Add mushrooms, onions, water chestnuts, and bamboo shoots. Stir often for about 4 minutes. Add the tofu, which has been rinsed and cut into small cubes. Stir the ingredients until the mushrooms and onions are nearly done. Stir in the oyster sauce. Serve over rice. Serves 4.

TOFU VEGETABLE QUICHE

½ pound tofu
¼ cup raw cashew nuts, washed
½ cup water
1 teaspoon Italian seasoning
Pinch garlic powder
1 teaspoon salt
2 tablespoons cornstarch or
    arrowroot powder
2 tablespoons olive oil (optional)

1 green pepper, diced
1 cup sliced broccoli or other
    vegetable, such as spinach or 1
    cup fresh mushrooms, sliced
½ cup canned pimiento,
    chopped
1 small onion, diced
½ cup bread crumbs, lightly oiled
    and seasoned

In blender or food processor blend until smooth the tofu, cashews, water, Italian seasoning, garlic powder, salt, and cornstarch. Sauté the remaining ingredients in the olive oil or you may use water. Add tofu mixture to sautéed vegetables and mix well. Put into prepared casserole, sprinkle crumbs on top. Bake 35 minutes at 350°. Serves 4.

⚜

SCRAMBLED TOFU

1 block (1 lb.) tofu, drained
1 teaspoon oil
1 tablespoon onion powder or ½
    cup sautéed onion
1 tablespoon soy sauce
½ teaspoon salt (use 1 teaspoon if
    soy sauce not used)

⅛-¼ teaspoon turmeric
1 teaspoon poultry seasoning
2 tablespoons textured vegetable
    protein (TVP) bacon bits
2 teaspoons yeast flakes

Stir the oil and all of the seasonings together in skillet and stir well to mix. Add tofu that has been broken up and coarsely mashed with fork. Mix thoroughly with the seasonings and heat. Serve like scrambled eggs. Serves 4.

FRESH STEWED TOMATO SAUCE & PASTA

1 tablespoon margarine
1 small onion, chopped
½ green pepper, chopped
1½ teaspoons garlic powder
¼ teaspoon pepper

1½ teaspoons Italian seasoning—
or to taste
2 pounds tomatoes, peeled
4-serving amount of pasta
¼ cup Parmesan cheese, grated

In large skillet, over medium heat, melt margarine and cook onions and green pepper until tender. Mash tomatoes, then add to skillet with remaining ingredients, bring to a boil, then simmer 30 minutes. Boil pasta until done, rinse in hot water. Serve tomato sauce over pasta, sprinkle with Parmesan cheese. Cooked ground turkey may be added to sauce for variation—also chopped mushrooms. Serves 4.

⚜

SPAGHETTI WITH BROCCOLI

1 bunch broccoli
4 small red tomatoes (about ½
    pound)
½ pound spaghetti
2 tablespoons olive oil
1 tablespoon garlic, finely minced
Pepper to taste, if desired

¼ teaspoon dried hot red pepper
flakes
½ cup evaporated skim milk
½ cup fresh basil, finely chopped
2 tablespoons Parmesan cheese,
grated

Cut broccoli into 1-2 inch pieces (makes about 4 cups). Cut tomatoes into ¼-inch cubes (makes about 1½ cups). Bring to boil enough water to cover broccoli and cook about 2 minutes. Drain. Cook and drain spaghetti.

In skillet, heat oil, add garlic, and cook until wilted. Add tomatoes and cook, stirring, about 1 minute. Add broccoli and pepper to taste. Add spaghetti, pepper flakes, milk, basil, and toss while bringing mixture barely to a boil. Remove from heat and sprinkle with cheese. Toss briefly and serve. Serves 6.

BROCCOLI-STUFFED SHELLS

3 cups broccoli florets
1 container (15 oz.) part-skim
    ricotta cheese
1 egg and 2 egg whites
2 tablespoons grated Parmesan
    cheese

¼ teaspoon black pepper
½ teaspoon nutmeg
½ teaspoon oregano
24 jumbo pasta shells, cooked
3 cups tomato sauce

Steam or boil broccoli florets until crunchy tender. Allow to cool. Mince florets, either with a sharp knife or in the base of a food processor fitted with a steel blade. Combine minced broccoli with ricotta, eggs, parmesan, pepper, nutmeg, and oregano, and stir until well combined. Stuff each cooked shell with about 1 tablespoon of the ricotta-broccoli mixture. Serves 8.

⚜

VEGETABLE-STUFFED GREEN PEPPERS

4 medium green peppers
1 tablespoon margarine
2 cups zucchini, chopped
1 cup mushrooms, chopped
½ cup onions, chopped
1 clove garlic, minced

1½ teaspoons fresh basil, chopped
    or ½ teaspoon dry
¼ teaspoon salt
¼ teaspoon pepper
½ cup plain croutons

Cut tops off green peppers. Remove membranes and seeds. Steam peppers for a few minutes. If you prefer green peppers crisp, omit this step. Preheat oven to 350°. In a skillet, saute zucchini, mushrooms, onions, garlic, and basil in margarine. Add salt and pepper. Cook uncovered over medium heat, stirring, until liquid has evaporated (about 10 minutes). Stir in croutons. Spoon vegetable mixture into peppers. Place in a 1½-quart baking dish. Bake, covered, about 15 minutes. Uncover and bake 5 more minutes. Serves 4.

DESSERTS

Give fruit and fruit desserts the place they deserve. Poached fruit, compotes, and fruit salad can appropriately end an elegant meal. Baked fruits are good as well. For a wholesome end to a meal, serve fresh strawberries with vanilla low fat yogurt.

Reserve baked desserts for special occasions. If you want to bake a dessert, use low fat ingredients only. Be pleased that you have mastered the art of low fat cooking to the ultimate—desserts.

BANANA-STRAWBERRY DELIGHT

2 ripe medium-size bananas
½ cup evaporated skim milk,
   chilled

½ teaspoon vanilla
1 cup strawberries, frozen and
   unsweetened

Peel bananas, cut into chunks. Freeze, covered, until firm. In blender or food processor, combine milk, bananas, and vanilla. Blend until smooth. Add strawberries a few at a time and blend until smooth. Garnish with sliced strawberries and serve at once. Serves 4.

⚜

BARTLETT BRUNCH COMPOTE

3 fresh pears
2 oranges, peeled and sliced
1 small cantaloupe, cut into
   chunks
½ pound grapes, halved and
   seeded

1 cup canned apricots
3 tablespoons sugar
3 tablespoons orange or
   pineapple juice

Peel, core, and slice pears into wedges. Combine pears, oranges, cantaloupe, and grapes. Drain apricots; puree until smooth in blender or food processor. Combine in small saucepan with sugar; heat until sugar dissolves. Add juice. Chill. Pour over fruit and toss lightly to coat. Serve chilled in individual serving dishes. Serves 6-8.

SPARKLING CHERRY GEL

2 cups pitted and chopped sweet
    cherries
½ cup water

1 package (3 oz.) raspberry gelatin
½ orange, chopped

It takes about 3 cups pitted cherries to make 2 cups chopped. Chop orange, skin and all, with fine blade or blender. Combine cherries and water in a 2-quart saucepan. Bring to a boil and cook 2 minutes. Remove from heat and blend in the gelatin until dissolved. Add chopped orange. Pour into mold or 8 x 8 glass dish. Serves 4 to 6.

🌿

PUMPKIN CHIFFON PUDDING

2 teaspoons gelatin
1 egg
⅔ cup pumpkin, cooked and
    strained

1¼ ounces skim or low fat milk
¼ teaspoon cinnamon
¼ teaspoon nutmeg
½ teaspoon sugar

Soften gelatin in 2 tablespoons of cold water. Separate egg. Beat yolk slightly and add to it the milk, pumpkin, spices, and sugar. Cook and stir over hot water until thick. Add gelatin and cool. Add a pinch of salt to egg white and whip until stiff. Fold into cool pumpkin mixture. Chill in refrigerator several hours before serving. Garnish with plain low fat yogurt mixed with a little sugar and vanilla. Serves 2-3.

PRUNE WHIP

1 cup pitted prunes, mashed
⅓ cup sugar
½ teaspoon lemon juice

½ teaspoon grated lemon rind
¼ teaspoon cinnamon
1 egg white

Cook prunes and sugar to consistency of marmalade. Add lemon juice, lemon rind, and cinnamon. Cool. Beat egg white very stiff. Fold into prune mixture. Chill. Serves 3 to 4.

STRAWBERRY YOGURT FROST

1 package (10 oz.) frozen, sweetened strawberries, sliced
1 cup low fat plain yogurt

⅓ cup instant nonfat dry milk
¾ cup water
1 teaspoon vanilla

Cut frozen block of strawberries in half. Place yogurt, nonfat dry milk, water, strawberries, and vanilla in blender container. Cover and process on high speed until smooth. Makes 3½ cups.

SORBET

2 cups fresh or frozen fruit (raspberries, strawberries, bananas, melon balls)
2 tablespoons powdered sugar

2 tablespoons liqueur (Kirsch, apricot brandy, etc.)
1 tablespoon plain low fat yogurt, if desired

Combine frozen fruit, sugar, and liqueur in food processor and blend to desired consistency. Serve immediately. Garnish with fresh mint and serve with plain low fat yogurt. Serves 4.

INSTANT SORBET

¼ cup low fat yogurt
2 egg whites
3 cups frozen fruit cut in small
   pieces (don't bother cutting
   small berries)

1-3 teaspoons sugar (depending
   on sweetness of fruit)
1-2 teaspoons lemon or lime juice

Place yogurt, egg whites, and juice in food processor; blend briefly. With processor running, gradually add frozen fruit until sorbet is formed (about 2 or 3 minutes). Serves 6.

❧

BAKED APPLES WITH MERINGUE

4 Rome Beauty apples
2-inch piece of vanilla bean
¼ cup sugar
½ cup water
2 egg whites
½ cup confectioners' sugar

4 teaspoons almonds or filberts,
   chopped

Garnish:
Strawberries

Peel and core apples. Put the apples and the piece of vanilla bean in a baking dish just large enough to hold them. Sprinkle the apples with sugar. Pour water into dish and bake at 375° for 35-40 minutes or until they are tender.

In a bowl beat egg whites until frothy. Beat in confectioners' sugar, 1 tablespoon at a time, and continue to beat until stiff. Sprinkle each apple with 1 teaspoon chopped nuts and top each apple with a portion of the meringue. Bake in 325° oven for 8-10 minutes or until lightly browned. Garnish with strawberries. Serves 4.

DESSERT MERINGUES

4 egg whites
½ teaspoon vanilla
¼ teaspoon cream of tartar

¼ cup sugar, divided into thirds
2 tablespoons chocolate chips or
nuts

Have metal bowl, beaters, and egg whites at room temperature. Line baking sheets with parchment. Beat egg whites with vanilla and cream of tartar until stiff. Gradually add sugar, a third at a time, beating until stiff. Do not beat, but fold in chocolate chips or nuts. Do not overfold. Drop by spoonfuls on baking sheet. Bake at 250° for 40-50 minutes. Makes 2 dozen.

❧

APPLE CRISP

4 small Golden Delicious apples,
cored, pared, and cut into
¼-inch thick slices
3 tablespoons granulated sugar,
divided
1 tablespoon raisins
1 teaspoon lemon juice

¼ teaspoon cinnamon
⅓ cup plus 2 teaspoons all-
purpose flour
⅛ teaspoon double-acting baking
powder
2 tablespoons margarine

In medium-size bowl, combine apple slices, 1 tablespoon sugar, raisins, lemon juice, and ⅛ teaspoon cinnamon. Transfer to a 1-quart casserole dish; set aside.

Into small bowl sift together flour, baking powder, and remaining ⅛ teaspoon cinnamon; add remaining 2 tablespoons sugar and stir. With pastry blender, or 2 knives used scissors-fashion, cut in margarine until mixture resembles coarse meal. Sprinkle flour mixture over apples and bake at 375° until apples are tender, about 35 minutes. Serves 4.

LEMON VELVET

1 container (8 oz.) low fat lemon
  yogurt
1 can (6 oz.) frozen orange juice
  concentrate

2½ cups low fat milk
1 teaspoon vanilla

Blend and serve. Serves 4.

⚜

ORANGE WHIP CHEESECAKE

1 envelope plus 1 teaspoon
  unflavored gelatin
1 cup low fat milk
1 egg and 4 egg whites
1 pint small-curd low fat cottage
  cheese

1 teaspoon vanilla
1 teaspoon grated orange peel
Dash salt
⅓ cup sugar
8 orange slices, halved

Sprinkle gelatin over milk in top of double boiler. Beat egg yolk lightly and add to milk. Set over boiling water. Cook, stirring, for 5 minutes until gelatin dissolves and mixture thickens slightly. Remove from heat, and cool to room temperature. Add cottage cheese, turn into blender jar, cover, and blend until smooth. Turn out, stir in vanilla, orange peel, and salt. Cool until mixture begins to thicken. Beat egg whites to soft peaks. Gradually beat in sugar, beating to a soft meringue. Fold into cheese mixture and turn into 8-inch spring-form pan. Chill until firm, at least 4 hours. Top cheesecake with orange slices when served. Serves 8.

DICED APPLE CAKE

¼ cup oil
1 cup sugar
1 egg or 2 egg whites
1 cup flour
1 teaspoon baking soda

¼ teaspoon nutmeg
2 cups apples, diced, unpeeled
2 tablespoons nuts, chopped
½ cup raisins

Mix oil, sugar, and egg. Sift flour, soda, and nutmeg; add alternately with apples to the wet ingredients. Add nuts and raisins. Bake in 9 x 9 pan at 350° for 45 minutes.

⚜

WHOLE WHEAT PEAR PIE

4 to 5 winter pears
⅔ cup whole wheat flour,
    divided
½ cup sugar
1 teaspoon ground cinnamon,
    divided

2 tablespoons lemon juice
1 (9-inch) unbaked whole wheat
    pastry shell (recipe below)
¼ cup packed brown sugar
2 tablespoons soft margarine

Core and slice unpeeled pears; reserve 3 slices for garnish. Toss pears with 2 tablespoons whole wheat flour, sugar, ¼ teaspoon cinnamon, and lemon juice. Place in pie shell. Combine remaining ingredients, except pear slices, and sprinkle over top. Bake at 350° for 50 minutes. Garnish with reserved pear slices.

Whole Wheat Pastry:
Combine 1¼ cups whole wheat flour with 2 tablespoons sugar, 2 tablespoons oil, and 3 tablespoons skim or low fat milk; mix well. Mixture will be crumbly. Press into 9-inch pie tin. Serves 6.

BLUEBERRY MERINGUE PIE

1¼ cups graham cracker crumbs
¼ cup margarine
2 tablespoons sugar
4 egg whites
¼ cup sugar

½ teaspoon almond extract
¼ teaspoon salt
½ teaspoon cream of tartar
1½ cups fresh or frozen
  blueberries, rinsed and drained

In a bowl, mix crumbs, margarine, and sugar. Press mixture into the bottom and sides of an ungreased 9-inch pie plate. Bake shell at 375° for 10 minutes. Beat egg whites until stiff. Gradually add sugar in very small amounts, beating continuously after each addition. Alternately, add almond extract, salt, and cream of tartar, beating until thick and glossy. Carefully fold in blueberries, being careful not to break the berries. Pile blueberry meringue into cooled crust. With back of wet tablespoon, make swirl designs in meringue. Bake at 300° for about 15 minutes or just until top browns slightly. Let cool before cutting. Serves 8.

❧

CARROT CAKE

1 cup white flour
1 cup whole wheat flour
2 teaspoons baking powder
1½ teaspoons baking soda
½ teaspoon salt (or less)
3 teaspoons cinnamon
1 cup sugar

¾ cup oil
4 egg equivalents
2 cups carrots, grated
1 can (8½ oz.) crushed pineapple,
  drained
2 tablespoons nuts, chopped

Sift white flour, wheat flour, baking powder, baking soda, salt, and cinnamon together. Add sugar, oil, and egg equivalents and mix well. Add carrots, nuts, and pineapple. Pour batter into lightly greased 9 x 12 cake pan. Bake at 350° for 35-40 minutes.

OATMEAL CARROT BARS

¾ cup packed brown sugar
¼ cup shortening
1 egg
1 teaspoon vanilla
1½-2 cups carrots, shredded
1 cup whole wheat flour

1 teaspoon baking powder
¼ teaspoon salt
1 teaspoon cinnamon
½-¾ cup oatmeal
2 tablespoons wheat germ
½ cup raisins

Cream brown sugar, shortening, and egg in large bowl until smooth. Add vanilla and carrots. Set aside. Stir flour, baking powder, salt, and cinnamon together. Add to creamed mixture. Mix in oatmeal, wheat germ, and raisins. Bake in lightly greased 9 x 9 x 2 pan at 350° for 30-35 minutes. Cut into squares. Makes 2 dozen.

❧

APPLE GRAHAM CRISP

1 medium apple, sliced
1 graham cracker, crushed
1 teaspoon margarine

Sugar to taste
Cinnamon to taste

Put apple in individual serving dish. Sprinkle graham cracker and margarine over top of apple slices and bake at 350° until bubbly. Add sugar and cinnamon to taste. Serves 1.

STRAWBERRY PIE

1½ cups flour
⅓ cup oil
2-3 tablespoons cold water
4-6 tablespoons heated, strained
   apricot preserves or red
   currant jelly
1 egg + 2 egg whites

½ cup sugar
½ cup flour
1 cup skim milk
2 teaspoons vanilla extract
1-1¼ quart fresh strawberries,
   washed and hulled

To prepare pastry shell, pour oil into the flour in a mixing bowl. Stir with fork until the mixture looks like meal. Add water, one tablespoon at a time, mixing with fork. Stir until dough holds together and almost cleans the side of the bowl. Gather dough together with hands; press into ball. Refrigerate a few minutes to make dough easier to work; shape into a flattened round. Roll out dough between 2 pieces of waxed paper. Peel off top paper; turn dough onto pie pan. Remove second sheet; fit pastry into pan. Trim and flute edges with fork or fingers. Prick bottom and sides well. Bake at 475° for 12-15 minutes. Brush bottom of baked shell with 2-3 tablespoons apricot preserves or currant jelly to seal. Cool.

To prepare filling, combine egg mixture and sugar in a saucepan for 2-3 minutes. Beat in ½ cup flour. Bring milk to boil and gradually pour in a thin stream of droplets into flour mixture. Set over moderately high heat and stir, reaching all over bottom of pan. As sauce comes to boil it will get lumpy then smooth out as you beat it. After sauce reaches boil, turn heat to moderately low for 2-3 minutes to cook the flour. Remove from heat. Beat in vanilla extract. Cool. Spread filling over bottom of baked shell. Put largest strawberry in the center, stem end in the filling, and arrange others similarly in circles, graduating down in size. Spoon or paint over the remaining apricot or currant jelly. Serve cold. Serves 6.

Variations:
Substitute fresh raspberries; grapes, pears, peaches, or apricots poached in water and lemon juice, peeled and sliced; or any combination of fruit—and arrange as you desire.

PARTY CARROT CAKE

2 cups sugar
½ cup oil
1½ cups whole wheat flour
1½ cups white flour
2½ teaspoons baking soda
2½ teaspoons cinnamon

½ teaspoon salt
2 cups shredded carrots
2 teaspoons vanilla
1 can (11 oz.) mandarin oranges,
    undrained
5 egg whites

Preheat oven to 350°. In large bowl, combine all cake ingredients. Beat 2 minutes at high speed. Pour into lightly oiled 9x13 inch pan. Bake 50-60 minutes or until wooden pick inserted in center comes out clean and cake pulls away from sides of pan. Cool. Cake can be removed from pan after 30 minutes.

♣

PINTO FIESTA CAKE

1 cup sugar
¼ cup margarine
2 egg whites, lightly beaten
2 cups cooked pinto beans,
    mashed, or vegetarian refried
    beans
1 cup flour
1 teaspoon baking soda

1 teaspoon cinnamon
½ teaspoon cloves
½ teaspoon allspice
2 cups diced raw apples
1 cup raisins
¼ cup chopped walnuts
2 teaspoons vanilla

Preheat oven to 375°. Cream sugar and margarine, add beaten egg whites. Add mashed beans. Mix well. Sift all dry ingredients, including spices, together and add to sugar mixture. Add apples, raisins, walnuts, and vanilla. Pour into lightly oiled 10-inch tube or bundt cake pan and bake for 45 minutes. Serves 16.

COCOA CAKE

1½ cups flour
1 cup sugar
1 teaspoon baking soda
3 tablespoons cocoa powder

3 tablespoons oil
1 teaspoon vanilla
1 tablespoon vinegar
1 cup cold water

Preheat oven to 350°. Sift dry ingredients together. Pour the liquid ingredients over the dry ingredients and stir until smooth. If making cupcakes, turn into 12 paper-lined muffin tins and bake for 25-30 minutes. For a cake, bake in ungreased 9-inch square pan for 35 minutes. Cool. Makes 12 cupcakes. Cake serves 9.

⚜

CREPES

1 cup nonfat milk
1 cup unbleached flour
1 large egg or 2 egg whites

1 teaspoon margarine
Vanilla low fat yogurt

Put in blender and mix well. Heat a 7- or 8-inch crepe pan or nonstick skillet with sloping edges. Melt margarine in pan. Add 2 tablespoons of batter to the hot pan and tip pan gently so that the batter completely covers the bottom. Cook the crepe over moderately high heat for 30-40 seconds or until the bottom of the crepe is lightly browned. Flip the crepe and cook for 15 seconds. Flip the crepe onto waxed paper. Repeat until all crepes are cooked, lightly oiling the pan each time if it is a nonstick pan. To fill each crepe, spread a tablespoon of vanilla low fat yogurt down the middle and roll up. Or serve with Light "Custard" Sauce. Makes 6.

BABA AU RHUM (SAVARIN)

2 packages active dry yeast
1 cup skim milk, lukewarm
4 cups white flour
6 egg whites
2 teaspoons sugar
½ teaspoon salt

5 tablespoons margarine

Rum Syrup:
2 cups sugar
2 cups water
1 cup rum

Dissolve yeast in lukewarm milk. In a large bowl, mix flour, egg whites, and dissolved yeast. The dough should be smooth. Cover and let rise for at least 1 hour and until the dough has doubled in volume. Melt margarine and add with sugar and salt to the dough. Mix well. It will be a soft, sticky dough. Oil a 12-cup mold (a ring mold works well) or a bundt cake pan. Put the dough in the pan to fill about halfway to the top. Let rise again for 1-2 hours. Bake in a 375° oven. If the top starts to become too brown cover for awhile with foil. Bake 30 minutes or until "baba" pulls away from sides of pan. Unmold while still warm and allow to cool. To make rum syrup, dissolve sugar in water. Bring to a boil and simmer for about 5 minutes, then add rum. Put "baba" back in the mold and pour the rum syrup over it, a tablespoon at a time, until all syrup is absorbed. Unmold and serve with Light "Custard" Sauce, strawberry or raspberry sauce, or any sauce of your choice. Makes 24 servings.

YOGURT SMOOTHIE

½ cup raspberries or hulled
   strawberries
⅔ cup plain low fat yogurt

1 large banana, cut in thirds
¼ cup nonfat or low fat milk, or
   apple juice

Place all ingredients in blender container and blend until smooth. Pour into 2 tall glasses. Serves 2.

LIGHT "CUSTARD" SAUCE

4 tablespoons granulated sugar
1 egg + 3 egg whites
1 teaspoon cornstarch

1¾ cup skim milk
1 teaspoon vanilla extract

In a 3-quart mixing bowl, gradually beat sugar into egg mixture until pale yellow. Heat milk to boiling point. Beat cornstarch into egg mixture and slowly pour boiling milk into mixture in a steady stream of droplets. Pour into medium-size saucepan. Set over moderate heat stirring constantly with wooden spoon until sauce thickens enough to coat spoon with creamy layer. Beat, off heat, to cool. Add vanilla to cool, stirring frequently. Cover, chill, serve. Makes 2½-3 cups.

⚘

BANANA MILKSHAKE

1 medium banana
½ cup low fat evaporated milk
½ cup skim milk

¼ teaspoon vanilla
2 scoops low fat frozen vanilla
  yogurt or ice milk

Peel banana, cut into 1-inch pieces, and wrap in aluminum foil. Freeze. In a blender container mix milks, vanilla, and banana. Blend until smooth. Pour into 2 tall glasses. Top each with scoop of frozen yogurt. Serves 2.

POACHED PEARS IN WINE

8 ripe, firm pears (Bosc are best)
3 cups red Burgundy wine
3 cups water
2 tablespoons lemon juice
4 whole cloves
1 cup granulated sugar

2 sticks or 1 teaspoon cinnamon
Acidulated water: 2 tablespoons
  lemon juice in 4 cups cold
  water
⅓ cup slivered almonds, to
  decorate

Peel pears and, using a small sharp knife, carefully remove the core from the bottoms, leaving the top stems intact. Drop pears in acidulated water to prevent discoloration. Place wine, water, lemon juice, cloves, and sugar in a saucepan. Heat to boiling. Drop in drained pears and let the syrup return to a boil. Turn down the heat and simmer uncovered for 12-15 minutes or until pears are firm but easily pierced with a knife. If pears are not completely immersed in the syrup, turn them from time to time during cooking so they will color evenly. Allow pears to cool in the syrup. Drain, reserving the syrup. Boil down syrup until it measures 1 cup. Serve pears in individual dishes with syrup spooned over them and a light "custard" sauce. Sprinkle with slivered almonds. Serves 8.

❧

STRAWBERRY MILKSHAKE

1 cup fresh or frozen strawberries
1 cup low fat evaporated milk
1 tablespoon lemon juice

2 scoops low fat frozen strawberry
  or lemon yogurt, or sherbet
Fresh mint to decorate

In a blender container combine milk, lemon juice, and strawberries. Blend until smooth. Pour into 2 tall glasses. Top each with one scoop of frozen yogurt or sherbet. Decorate with fresh mint. Serves 2.

RECIPE CONTRIBUTORS

❧

Numerous organizations and Oregon volunteers offered their recipes for inclusion in *Simply Nutritious!* Some recipes came in anonymously. All contributors deserve our thanks.

American Heart Association Cookbook—Chuck's Chicken & Vegetables, Mock Sour Cream

Ruth Anderson—Lunch Salad, Molded Salad, Apple Graham Crisp, Pumpkin Chiffon Pudding

Arlene Anibal—Scrambled Tofu, Tofu Vegetable Quiche, Best Corn-Oat Waffles

Sabine Artaud-Wild, R.D.— Strawberry Milkshake, Banana Milkshake, Apple Butter

Delores Atiyeh—Tabooley

Congressman Les AuCoin—Onion Wine Soup

Susie Bamer—Natural Bran Muffins

Carol Berkley, "It's Your Party" Caterers—Fancy & Fresh Cocktail Potatoes

Eve Black—Low Calorie Spinach Dip, Harry's Bagels

Connie Bondi—Three-Bran Muffins

Margie Boule—Chinese Chicken Salad

Peggy Carey—Hummus, Mimi's Tuna Salad, Linguine with Clam Sauce

Marie M. Carlson—Polynesian Dinner

Joan Corcoran—Dilly Tuna Dip

Emily Crumpacker, Food Consultant—Wild Rice Salad, Fillet of Sole with Garlic & Spinach

Shirley J. Cuff—Baked Chicken with Mushrooms & Onions

Francis Dietrichs—Cranberry Relish Salad

Kathleen Drewelow—Louisiana Chicken Casserole

Evelyn Dwigans—Friendship Bean Soup

Judy Dyer, R.D.—Black Beans & Rice

Prudence Dyer—Turkey (Chicken) Stir-Fry

Janet Earhart—Chicken Breasts with Sherry

Judith Poxson Fawkes—Minestrone Di Oregon Soup
Nancy Frazeur, R.D.—Low Calorie Savory Salad Dressing
LouAnn Frisch, R.D.—Broccoli with Orange Sauce

Beverly Galen—Chestnut Dressing, Spinach-Wrapped Chicken with Dip,
    Peach Chutney, Pita Bread, Chicken & Prunes, Baked Apples with
    Meringue, Prune Whip
Dr. William Galen—Dr. Galen's Breakfast Choice
Tracy Garrett—Cold Asparagus with Walnuts, Whole Wheat Raisin Bread,
    Carrot Bread, Baked Orange Roughy, Lemon Dill Rice, Oven-Fried Potatoes,
    Sorbet
Shirley Gittelsohn—Stir-Fried Fish Dinner
Gayle Gray—Buttermilk Quick Bread, Buttermilk Corn Bread, Mexican
    Vegetables
Esther Grenley—Hayden's Chicken Delight

Cheryl Hansen—Cheryl's Rainbow Salad
Helen Bernhard Bakery—Bran Muffins

Jan and Peter Jacobsen—Fresh Stewed Tomato Sauce & Pasta
Helen E. Johnson—100% Whole Wheat Bread
Linda Jones, I. Magnin & Co.—Chicken Caruso

Dorothy S. Kien—Fruited Bran Muffins, Crepes
Ethel Kinsley—Spiced Cauliflower, Banana-Strawberry Delight
Bonnie Kirby—Dessert Meringues
Ann Kracke—Whole Wheat Sunflower Muffins
Margery Krueger—Millet Cereal

Lorna Leong—Elk with Fresh Broccoli
Katherine Lite—Baked Chicken, Diced Apple Cake
Matthew E. Littau—Stir-Fried Mushrooms & Tofu

Marvel's Health Store—Chili
Carolyn Medean—No-Knead Wheat Bread
Audrey Mills—Barley Soup
Margaret Mills—Fresh Fruit Salad
Anne Myers—Irish Soda Bread

Marilyn J. Naish—Oatmeal Carrot Bars
Kim Nelson—Seafood Casserole

The New American Diet Cookbook—Antipasto, Chili Bean Salad, Sunshine Spinach Salad, Low Fat Granola, Fillet of Fish Florentine, Broccoli with Rice, Herbed Brussels Sprouts, Dill Cabbage, Vegetable-Stuffed Green Peppers, Carrot Cake, Strawberry Pie, Party Carrot Cake, Pinto Fiesta Cake, Cocoa Cake. Recipes developed by Sabine Artaud-Wild for *The New American Diet Cookbook*—Ratatouille Provencale, Baba Au Rhum (Savarin), Poached Pears in Wine, Light "Custard" Sauce

Margery M. O'Brien—Baked Trout in Wine
Mildred Olson—Sparkling Cherry Gel
Sandy Olson—Chili for a Crowd
Oregon Beef Council—Hearty Taco Soup
Oregon Blueberry Growers Association—Blueberry Meringue Pie
Oregon Dairy Council—Spiced Cheese, Yogurt/Honey/Sesame Dip, Strawberry Yogurt Frost, Orange Whip Cheesecake, Lemon Velvet
Oregon Dairy Products Commission—Spinach Salad with Curry Yogurt Dressing
Oregon Filbert Commission—Frontier Hazelnut Vegetable Pie, Hazelnut Broccoli
Oregon Fryer Commission—Chicken Salad A La Yogurt, Super Low Calorie Chicken, Lemon Chicken, Chicken Creole, Chicken Florentine, Quick Chick Skillet, Chickenburgers, Crispy Oven-Fried Lemon Chicken, Chicken Breasts with Apricots & Avocado
Oregon Potato Commission—Salmon-Stuffed Potatoes
Oregon Processed Prune and Plum Growers Commission—Chicken Breasts with Curried Fruit
Oregon Turkey Improvement Association—Turkey Polynesian
Oregon, Washington, California Pear Bureau—Pear Shrimp Salad, Bartlett Brunch Compote, Whole Wheat Pear Pie, Pear Relish
Oregon Wheat Commission—Bulgur Cabbage Salad, Carrot Sandwich Bread, Sourdough Starter
Otter Trawl Commission of Oregon—Perch Piquant, Northwest Cioppino

Senator Bob Packwood—Cranberry Salad
Vera Payne—Oatmeal Bread
Nancy Pearson—Soy Salad Dressing, Tuna Macaroni Salad
Wanda Phipps, Multnomah County Extension Service—Portuguese Fisherman Stew, Spaghetti with Broccoli
John and Louise Piacentini—Split Pea Vegetable Soup

Jane Reed—Tuna & Green Bean Casserole
Martha Rutherford, Panache Caterers—Cold Cucumber Soup, Pasta Broccoli Salad, Chicken with Cumin & Ginger

Anita Schacher—Springtime Vegetable Soup
Arlene Schnitzer—Arlene's Mother's Sole
Doris Schnitzer—Vegetable Dip
Lois Schnitzer—Spinach Orange Salad, Banana Prawn Curry
Mildred Schnitzer—Chicken Sukiyaki
Susan Schnitzer—Eggplant Dip, Baked Halibut, Tuna Loaf, Alpine Rice, Vegetable Casserole
Doris Schwab—Zucchini Rice Casserole, Marinated Broccoli
Nancy Sideras—Yia Yia's Mumbaldi
Sandy Smith—Marvelous Meatloaf
Nancy Strope—Glazed Carrots

Dan and Kathleen Taggart, Kitchen Kaboodle—Taggart's Spicy Chicken with Cashews
Marcelle Tebo—Pickled Green Beans
Nancy Tonkin—Lemony Chicken Breasts

Georgia Vareldzis—Fassolada (Greek Bean Soup)
Pat Vincent—Marinated Vegetables

Virginia Wasmund—Molded Fruit Summer Salad
Diane Waters—Fruited Chicken Salad
Weight Watchers of Oregon, Inc.—Sherried Mushroom Soup, Poultry in a Pocket-To-Go, Stuffed Flounder Fillets, Creamed Brussels Sprouts, Apple Crisp

Evelyn Zurow—Instant Sorbet

FURTHER NOTES ON PREVENTION

⚜

Simply Nutritious! is a tool you can use to improve your health and reduce your risk of getting cancer. This is exciting news for both the general public and the medical community. It further places the final responsibility for individual health with the individual. You can have a significant effect upon development and course of diseases in your life—by the lifestyle decisions you make and by the level of personal awareness you maintain about your body and its proper functioning.

Cancer does not just appear one day, but develops over a period of weeks, months, or years. Many factors, including family history, personal habits, workplace hazards, diet, and carcinogens in the environment may play a role in the development of cancer. (See the chapter titled Research.) So simple prevention is not enough. You must be aware of the risk factors created by your family history or your exposure to possible carcinogens. You should also be aware of the symptoms of diseases, including cancer, and communicate changes or irregularities in your body to a physician. Critical to your health maintenance plan are establishing an open, working relationship with your physician and routine office visits.

To make *Simply Nutritious!* a more complete tool for controlling cancer in your life, we have included this section on primary and secondary prevention. Use the information here, and if you have further questions, contact your physician or the American Cancer Society.

Our goal is to help you and those you love live a long and happy life free from cancer.

Leroy Groshong, M.D.
Surgical Oncologist
Past President, American Cancer Society,
Oregon Division, Inc.

PRIMARY PREVENTION

Nutrition

See the American Cancer Society Interim Dietary Guidelines set forth earlier in this book.

Smoking

Cigarette smoking is responsible for 85% of lung cancer cases among men and 75% among women. If the number of smokers was reduced by half, 75,000 lives would be saved each year. Smoking accounts for about 30% of all cancer deaths. Smokeless tobaccos are highly habit forming and result in increased risk factors for cancers of the mouth, larynx, throat, and esophagus.

Alcohol

Oral cancer and cancers of the larynx, throat, esophagus, and liver occur more frequently among heavy drinkers of alcohol.

Sunlight

Almost all of the 400,000 cases of non-melanoma skin cancer developed each year in the U.S. are considered to be sun-related. Recent epidemiological evidence shows that sun exposure is a major factor in the development of melanoma and that the incidence increases for those living near the equator.

Radiation

Excessive exposure to X-ray can increase cancer risk. Today, most medical X-rays are adjusted to deliver the lowest dose possible without sacrificing image quality.

Estrogens

For mature women, there are certain risks associated with estrogen treatment to control menopausal symptoms, including an increased risk of endometrial cancer. However, estrogen can be given safely under careful physician control.

Occupational

Exposure to a number of industrial agents (including nickel, chromate, asbestos, and vinyl chloride) increases risk. The risk factor greatly increases when combined with smoking.

SECONDARY PREVENTION

Colorectal

The American Cancer Society recommends three tests for the early detection of colon and rectal cancer in people without symptoms. The digital rectal examination, performed by a physician during an office visit, should be performed every year after the age of 40; the stool blood test is recommended every year after 50; and the proctosigmoidoscopy examination should be carried out every 3-5 years after the age of 50 following two annual examinations with negative results.

Pap Test

For the average risk person, a Pap test is recommended annually until two consecutive satisfactory tests are negative, and then once every three years. The Pap test is highly effective in detecting cancer of the uterine cervix, but is less effective in detecting endometrial cancer.

Breast Cancer Detection

The American Cancer Society recommends the monthly practice of breast self-examination (BSE) by women 20 years and older as a routine good health habit. Physical examination of the breast should be done every three years from ages 20-39 and then every year. The Society recommends a mammogram every year for asymptomatic women age 50 and over, and a baseline mammogram between ages 35 and 39. Women 40-49 should have mammography every 1 or 2 years depending on physical and mammographic findings.

FURTHER READING

࿇

Calorie Counters

Calories and Carbohydrates. Barbara Kraus. Signet (New American Library), New York, 1975.

The Dictionary of Sodium, Fats, and Cholesterol. Barbara Kraus. Grosset and Dunlap, New York, 1974.

Food Composition

Food Values of Portions Commonly Used, 13th ed. Jean A. T. Pennington and Helen Nichols Church. Harper and Row, New York, 1980.

Nutrition

Jane Brody's Nutrition Book. Jane Brody. W. W. Norton, New York, 1981 and Bantam, New York, 1982.

Nutrition/Cookbooks

The American Heart Association Cookbook, 4th ed. David McKay Company, Inc., New York, 1984.

The Best of the Family Heart Kitchens. S. L. Connor, W. E. Connor, N. Becker, et al. Oregon Health Sciences University, Portland, OR, 1981.

The Family Health Cookbook. Alice White and Society for Nutrition Education. David McKay Company, Inc., New York, 1980.

The F-Plan Diet. Audrey Eyton. Bantam, New York, 1984.

The High Fiber Cookbook. Pamela Westland. Arco Publishing Inc., New York, 1982.

Jane Brody's Good Food Book: Living the High Carbohydrate Way. Jane Brody. W. W. Norton, New York, 1985.

Laurel's Kitchen: A Handbook for Vegetarian Cookery & Nutrition. Laurel Robertson, Carol Flinders, and Bronwen Godfrey. Nilgiri Press, Berkeley, 1977.

Lean Cuisine. Barbara Gibbons. Harper and Row, New York, 1979.

Lose Weight Naturally Cookbook. Sharon Claessens. Rodale Press, Emmaus, PA, 1986.

The Low Fat Lifestyle. Valerie Parker and Ronda Gates. LFL Associates, Lake Oswego, OR, 1984.

The New American Diet. Sonja L. and William E. Connor. Simon and Schuster, New York, 1986.

Magazines/Journals

Nutrition Action. Center for Science in the Public Interest, 1755 S Street NW, Washington, DC 20009.

INDEX

ᴪ

Fruits, 14
   amount in diet, 13
   in balanced diet, 14-15
   fat content of, 14, 20
   guidelines on, 8, 9
   as snacks, 43
   as source of fiber, 24, 25, 26
   as source of vitamins A and C, 27,
      28
Frying and fried foods, 12, 29

Grains, 15
   amount in diet, 13, 15
   in balanced diet, 15
   used in breads and cereals, 90-101
   fat content of, 20
   recipes using, 68, 78, 83, 85
   as source of fiber, 24, 25, 26
Granola,
   recipe for, 101
   as snack, 45
Gravies, 38

Health foods, 45, 51

Imitation foods, 29

Labeling on foods, 19, 29, 30, 35, 45
Legumes, 15; *also see* Vegetables
   amount in diet, 15
   in balanced diet, 15
   as protein source, 15, 17
   recipes using, 60, 65, 68, 70, 71, 74,
      82, 108
   as source of fiber, 24, 25, 26

Light foods, 29
Low calorie foods, 29
Luncheon meats, 16, 30
Lunch, brownbag, 48

Mayonnaise,
   fat content of, 23
   imitation, 55
   real, 41, 55
Meats,
   cooking methods, 28
   frying, 12, 29
   guideline on, 10
   preserved, 29, 30
   recipes using, 74, 115, 140, 142
   reducing use, 28, 42, 54
   selecting, 16, 30, 34
   as protein source, 14, 16, 28, 30

Milk products; also see Dairy
   Products
   fat content of, 21, 30
   reducing use, 28, 54
   selecting, 31
Minerals; *also see* Calcium
   in balanced diet, 15-17
Muffins, recipes for, 95, 98, 99
Mustard family vegetables, 9, 14, 103

Nuts and seeds, 15
   amount in diet, 16
   in balanced diet, 15
   fat content of, 20
   as protein source, 15
   as snacks, 45

Obesity, guideline on, 7
Organ meats, 34, 54

Pancakes, recipe for, 100
Poultry, 16; *also see* Chicken
    cooking methods, 38
    fat content of, 22
    portions of, 17, 30, 54
    as protein source, 16, 17, 28, 30
    recipes using, 61, 111-126, 139
Protein,
    amount in diet, 14, 16
    amounts in some foods, 17
    animal, in balanced diet, 16
    reducing animal sources of, 16, 28
    selecting animal sources, 34
    shopping tips for animal sources,
      30

Reduced calorie foods, 29
Reducing fat intake, *see* Fats and Oils
Restaurant foods, *see* Eating Out Tips

Salad dressing, 75
    recipes for, 49, 50, 53, 65, 66, 67, 69
Salads, 75
    recipes for, 63-73
Salt (sodium),
    reduced in recipes, 54
    risks of, 54
Selenium, 11
Shopping to reduce fat, 29-35
Snacks and snacking, 23-24, 43-45
Sodium, *see* Salt
Soups, recipes for, 54-61

Sour cream,
    fat content of, 21
    substitute, recipe for, 64
Steakhouses, 49
Stocks and broths, 38-39
Substitutions, cooking and baking, 42-43
Sugars,
    reduced in recipes, 55

Simply Nutritious! is the result of a collaboration among staff and volunteers for the American Cancer Society, Oregon Division, Inc., and editorial and graphic arts professionals. Susan Schnitzer chaired the committee; Philip Miller, Director of Crusade, represented ACS staff; Sabine M. Artaud-Wild, R.D., edited for content; Susan Page-York edited for structure and style; Patti Morris proofread; Susan Applegate designed the book and prepared it for printing; Mark Beach coordinated production.

The painting reproduced on the cover was donated by Portland artist Sally Haley whose work often depicts familiar domestic objects.

Simply Nutritious! committee members: Beverly Galen, Lindsay Galen, Ethel Kinsley, Kathrine Lite, Philip Miller, Margaret Mills, Sandy Olson, Cathy Rowland, Susan Schnitzer, Chair, Deanna Voytilla.

Type in this book is Cartier set 12/13½ by Irish Setter in Portland, Oregon. Printing and binding are by Publishers Press and Mountain States Bindery, both in Salt Lake City, Utah.

Simply Nutritious! Order Form

Please send _____ copies of *Simply Nutritious!* at $10.00 each plus
$1.50 postage and handling per copy. I enclose an additional donation of
$ _____ . Enclosed is my check or money order for $ _____ .

NAME _____

ADDRESS _____

CITY _____ STATE _____ ZIP _____

American Cancer Society, Nevada Division, Inc.
1325 E. Harmon
Las Vegas, NV 89119

Simply Nutritious! Order Form

Please send _____ copies of *Simply Nutritious!* at $10.00 each plus
$1.50 postage and handling per copy. I enclose an additional donation of
$ _____ . Enclosed is my check or money order for $ _____ .

NAME _____

ADDRESS _____

CITY _____ STATE _____ ZIP _____

American Cancer Society, Nevada Division, Inc.
1325 E. Harmon
Las Vegas, NV 89119

Simply Nutritious! Order Form

Please send _____ copies of *Simply Nutritious!* at $10.00 each plus
$1.50 postage and handling per copy. I enclose an additional donation of
$ _____ . Enclosed is my check or money order for $ _____ .

NAME _____

ADDRESS _____

CITY _____ STATE _____ ZIP _____

American Cancer Society, Nevada Division, Inc.
1325 E. Harmon
Las Vegas, NV 89119